T0075107

Navigating Communication with Seriously Ill Patients

Second Edition

When clinicians communicate effectively, patients retain more information, have higher trust, and a better quality of life. Such a patient-centered approach is the cornerstone of clinical care, and this book is an essential how-to guide on improving these skills.

Grounded in innovative and evidence-based methodology, perfected through over 20 years of teaching in the VitalTalk training program, content includes foundational communication skills, how to help patients plan for the future, what to do when you are really stuck, and strategies to work through conflicts with colleagues. In this updated edition, emphasis is placed on the roles privilege, race, and power play in the medical encounter, and new tools are provided to help clinicians navigate this landscape with greater self-awareness and sensitivity.

This practical guide is filled with skills and roadmaps, demonstrating how to be clearer when sharing information, more competent at understanding patient concerns, and more effective when making recommendations.

Robert M. Arnold, MD, FACP, FAAHPM, is Distinguished Service Professor of Medicine in the Division of General Internal Medicine and the Center for Bioethics and Health Law at the Icahn School of Medicine at Mount Sinai. He was the Past President of the American Society of Bioethics and Humanities (ASBH) as well as the American Academy of Hospice and Palliative Medicine (AAHPM). He has mentored both investigators and educators, and helped start VitalTalk, a nonprofit organization whose aim is to ensure that every seriously ill patient has clinicians who can talk about what matters most.

Anthony L. Back, MD, is Professor of Medicine at the University of Washington in Seattle. His research into patient–oncologist communication led to the founding of VitalTalk. His awards include the American Cancer Society (ACS) Pathfinder in Palliative Care Award and the American Society of Clinical Oncology Walther Cancer Foundation Palliative and Supportive Care Award.

Elise C. Carey, MD, FACP, FAAHPM, is Associate Professor of Medicine at Mayo Clinic in Rochester, Minnesota and Chair of Education & Faculty Development for the Mayo Clinic enterprise-wide Palliative Care Specialty Council. Dr. Carey currently serves on the Board of Directors of the American Academy of Hospice and Palliative Medicine and as a Strategic Partner and Distinguished Faculty with VitalTalk. She has been recognized nationally for her contributions to education and program development, including winning the Hastings Center Cunniff-Dixon Physician Award in 2014.

James A. Tulsky, MD, FACP, FAAHPM, is the Poorvu Jaffe Chair of the Department of Psychosocial Oncology and Palliative Care at Dana-Farber Cancer Institute, Chief of the Division of Palliative Medicine at Brigham and Women's Hospital, Professor of Medicine at Harvard Medical School, and a cofounder of VitalTalk. Dr. Tulsky has received multiple awards for his work devoted to improving the experience for patients living with serious illness including the ACS Pathfinder in Palliative Care Award and the AAHPM Award for Research Excellence.

Gordon J. Wood, MD, MSCI, FAAHPM, is Associate Professor of Medicine and Medical Education in the Section of Palliative Medicine at Northwestern University Feinberg School of Medicine. Dr. Wood currently serves as the Associate Director of the Education in Palliative and End-of-Life Care (EPEC) Program and as a Strategic Partner and Distinguished Faculty with VitalTalk. He has received multiple awards including being named an Inspiring Hospice and Palliative Medicine Leader Under 40 by the American Academy of Hospice and Palliative Medicine in 2014.

Holly Yang, MD MSHPEd, HMDC, FACP, FAAHPM, is the Scripps Health Co-Director of the University of California–San Diego/Scripps Health Hospice and Palliative Medicine Fellowship Program, and a Voluntary Associate Clinical Professor of Medicine at University of California, San Diego. She has been involved in interprofessional palliative care education nationally and internationally and has served as President of the American Academy of Hospice and Palliative Medicine. Dr. Yang is a Strategic Partner and Distinguished Faculty with VitalTalk.

Navigating Communication with Seriously Ill Patients

Balancing Honesty with Empathy and Hope

Second Edition

Robert M. Arnold

Icahn School of Medicine at Mount Sinai

Anthony L. Back

University of Washington

Elise C. Carey

Mayo Clinic

James A. Tulsky

Dana-Farber Cancer Institute

Gordon J. Wood

Northwestern University Feinberg School of Medicine

Holly B. Yang

Scripps Health

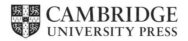

CAMBRIDGE
UNIVERSITY PRESS

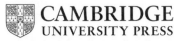

Shaftesbury Road, Cambridge CB2 8EA, United Kingdom

One Liberty Plaza, 20th Floor, New York, NY 10006, USA

477 Williamstown Road, Port Melbourne, VIC 3207, Australia

314–321, 3rd Floor, Plot 3, Splendor Forum, Jasola District Centre, New Delhi – 110025, India

103 Penang Road, #05–06/07, Visioncrest Commercial, Singapore 238467

Cambridge University Press is part of Cambridge University Press & Assessment,
a department of the University of Cambridge.

We share the University's mission to contribute to society through the pursuit of
education, learning and research at the highest international levels of excellence.

www.cambridge.org
Information on this title: www.cambridge.org/9781108925853

DOI: 10.1017/9781108921107

First edition © Anthony Back, Robert Arnold, and James Tulsky 2009

Second edition © Robert M. Arnold, Anthony L. Back, Elise C. Carey, James A. Tulsky, Gordon J. Wood,
and Holly B. Yang 2024

First published 2009
Second edition 2024

Printed in the United Kingdom by TJ Books Limited, Padstow Cornwall

A catalogue record for this publication is available from the British Library

Library of Congress Cataloging-in-Publication Data
Names: Carey, Elise C., author. | Back, Anthony. Mastering communication
with seriously ill patients.
Title: Navigating communication with seriously ill patients : balancing
honesty with empathy and hope / Robert M. Arnold [and 5 others].
Description: Second edition. | Cambridge, United Kingdom ; New York :
Cambridge University Press, 2024. | Preceded by Mastering communication
with seriously ill patients / Anthony Back, Robert Arnold, James Tulsky.
2009. | Includes bibliographical references and index.
Identifiers: LCCN 2023044504 | ISBN 9781108925853 (paperback) | ISBN
9781108921107 (ebook)
Subjects: MESH: Physician-Patient Relations | Critical Care | Terminally
Ill | Professional-Family Relations
Classification: LCC RT120.I5 | NLM W 62 | DDC 616.02/8–dc23/eng/20231101
LC record available at https://lccn.loc.gov/2023044504

ISBN 978-1-108-92585-3 Paperback

For Zeke Tulsky (1997–2023), who lived for human connection and instinctively understood the power of empathy to heal and to comfort. Like Zeke, in our work with patients may we always find the goodness in each person and the value of hearing their story.

"This book helps us to step away from our checklists and learn how to build genuine human connections with the people we are caring for."

Diane E. Meier, MD. Center To Advance Palliative Care. Professor, Department of Geriatrics and Palliative Medicine, Icahn School of Medicine at Mount Sinai

"Written by world-renowned educators, this expansive new edition will help clinicians not only understand the structure of compassionate serious illness communication but also the rationale behind it."

Vicki Jackson, MD, MPH. Blum Family Endowed Chair in Palliative Care. Chief, Division of Palliative Care and Geriatrics, Massachusetts General Hospital. Co-Director, Harvard Medical School Center for Palliative Care. Professor of Medicine, Harvard Medical School

"Every clinician committed to fostering meaningful connections with their patients and their families needs this book on their desk."

R. Sean Morrison, MD. Ellen and Howard C. Katz Professor and Chair. Brookdale Department of Geriatrics and Palliative Medicine.

"The updated *Navigating Communication with Seriously Ill Patients* presents foundational communication strategies along the trajectory of serious illness, now with critical attention to inclusiveness. It is an essential text for all who care for seriously ill patients of any age and life stage and their families."

Joanne Wolfe, MD MPH. Pediatric Palliative Care Physician. Chair, Department of Pediatrics, Massachusetts General Hospital. Chair, Department of Pediatrics, Brigham and Women's Hospital. Professor of Pediatrics, Harvard Medical School.

Contents

Preface

In 2009, when Tony, Bob, and James wrote the first edition of this book, we drew on a decade of experience studying and teaching communication, primarily within oncology. In the 14 years since, as medicine and the world have changed enormously, so has our approach to communication skills training. We've moved beyond only cancer care (Oncotalk) and created tailored courses such as Geritalk, Nephrotalk, and Cardiotalk to accommodate the full spectrum of serious illness. We've recognized that good communication depends on an interdisciplinary team and have sought to develop a far less physician-centered approach. We've learned from a now-robust literature on serious illness communication and incorporated wisdom from around the world on how to communicate best with patients and families. We've been profoundly affected by the long-needed awakening to the central role race and culture play in our society, including the delivery of health care, and have thought deeply about issues such as power and privilege in serious illness communication. And, perhaps most importantly, we created VitalTalk (in 2012) as a nonprofit vehicle to broadly disseminate communication skills teaching at a much larger scale. In doing so, we have trained more than 1,000 faculties who have, in turn, touched tens of thousands of learners around the globe. With the creation of digital learning tools and new pedagogical models we hope to reach countless more. In the process, we've also been deeply gratified by the power of the VitalTalk community that has arisen to support this work. The project has grown well beyond the three founders, and this edition was written together with Elise, Gordon, and Holly, who have been partners in our work since the early days of VitalTalk.

What Has Changed, and What Has Stayed the Same?

The last three years have brought a global pandemic, a huge shift toward care via telehealth, and, of course, a reckoning about health equity. The daily emails we receive from our health systems look radically different than just a few short years ago. The need for high-quality communication has become an even greater priority for many health systems as they see the kinds of skills we offer as part of the solution to their problems. During the height of the COVID-19 pandemic clinicians struggled to communicate empathically and effectively to patients making profound treatment choices, sometimes in the setting of true scarcity, and families unable to be with their desperately ill loved ones. And, as telehealth has boomed, so has the need to learn how to transmit empathy through a screen. Also, while race and culture have always played a role in health-care communication, many of us are now far more aware of the benefits and damage we can wield with our words.

VitalTalk has sought to respond to each of these challenges. Within weeks of the pandemic reaching our shores we produced the COVID Ready Communication Playbook to help clinicians with these difficult conversations. To our amazement, it was rapidly translated by our community into 25 languages. We adapted our face-to-face courses to be taught over a virtual platform and, in doing so, found ourselves teaching communication skills for virtual visits. We rewrote our cases and broadened our simulated patient actor pool to better represent the wide diversity of patients for whom we care. And we introduced anti-racist concepts into our mobile courses and new talking maps. Finally, we are excited to have just released a new mobile course entitled, "Building Connection: Practical Skills to Promote Racial Equity in Healthcare Communication."

We have emphasized this work too little in the past and we hope that our current efforts can begin to fill some of the gaps that currently exist in communication skills training. We are also aware that paying close attention to difference has always been at the heart of what we do at VitalTalk. The communication tools we promote are meant to create an environment in which every patient's needs are addressed and where care is driven by what matters most to the individual patient. When one patient's needs are not met, we all lose out.

So, over the past 14 years much has changed … and much has remained the same. Clinicians still care for patients confronting dreadful diagnoses that will change the course of their lives. They must still help them navigate these illnesses, cope with the outcomes, and, too frequently, make heart-wrenching decisions about treatment. And, too often, they still fall into familiar traps that lead to circular conversations, dissatisfied patients, and frustrated clinicians. The VitalTalk approach is about combining one's authentic self with evidence-based global communication skills and situation-specific talking maps to break these cycles and thereby to nurture meaningful conversations and healthy relationships. We also hope these tools will help with communication across differences, and when we see these opportunities, this book will point them out.

Who Is This Book For?

This book is for all clinicians who want to communicate better with seriously ill patients and their family members. We wrote the first edition with physicians in mind and yet some of our most positive feedback came from nurses, social workers, and others who found that these skills deeply resonated for them as well. Therefore, we enter this revision even more cognizant that patients receive the best care from an interdisciplinary team. Although some of the tools we discuss are most directly relevant to prescribing clinicians (typically Medical Doctors (MDs), Nurse Practitioners (NPs), and Physician Assistants (PAs)) who are the ones to usually guide patients through medical decision-making in advanced illness, everyone who sees patients should benefit from approaches that help defuse conflict, support patients, and learn from patients what matters most.

Since the first edition was published, many more readers will have had some communication training, and many more have been formally trained in palliative care. Therefore, for some, foundational concepts presented in this book, such as delivering serious news, may ring familiar. Others may be familiar with a great deal of the teaching in these pages. Recognizing that everyone has their learning edge, we've tried to shape this book so that all readers can find valuable take-home points, whether it is a refresher, engaging with an entirely new concept, or simply putting names to skills you already use in practice. By being better able to describe and deconstruct your own communication and that of your patients, families, and colleagues, we hope to help you enhance your own skills and teach others. And by doing so, we hope you can find deeper meaning in your work and even protect yourself against the burnout that comes from feeling powerless in the face of suffering.

What's in This Book?

In this book, we describe a variety of communication tools and "roadmaps" that you can use to find your way through difficult conversations. In our years of teaching learners of all backgrounds, we have found that many have either not seen a really good conversation, or they have not been able to identify what made the conversation work. Expert clinicians in action with patients can be so fluid, so seamless, so responsive, that they make great communication look easy. In fact, these master clinicians are collecting lots of data from the patients, drawing from a large repertoire of skills, and constantly readjusting their gestures and words. This master clinician could be you.

How Will This Book Help Me?

Adopting in your own practice the tools and roadmaps we've laid out will make you a better communicator. What do we mean by better? You'll be clearer about where your patients stand, more skillful at understanding their concerns, and more effective when you make recommendations. You'll be the kind of clinician that people want for their family and friends. And you'll develop a deeper sense of what matters to you in your clinical work because you will be talking to patients about what really matters to them.

However, a word of caution. The roadmaps are guides, not rules that must be followed. As you get more comfortable with serious illness communication, it is critical to integrate them into your personality so the result is genuine.

How Did We Develop This Book?

For over 25 years we have been teaching communication courses to students, trainees, and staff clinicians in what has come to be known as the VitalTalk method. Several of us have also been deeply involved in studying communication, audio-recording thousands of conversations, and observing what happens in actual practice. We have also learned from other investigators and master teachers. In fact, some of our greatest influences have come from unexpected places, including athletic coaches and elementary school educators. We've come to appreciate where clinicians typically get stuck, and the power of identifying key skills, providing roadmaps for conversations, and having people practice. We have been amazed at how learning a few key tools can change the way someone communicates. Listening to them talk about difficult topics with patients before and after training has been like observing completely different clinicians. Learners who have attended our courses tell us that these communication skills have changed how they approach patients, how they deal with emotional moments, and, most important, how they feel about their work.

Why Did We Write This Book?

Difficult patient encounters frustrate many of us daily. When we face demanding – sometimes tragic – situations, using communication skills that are "okay" is like riding a bike with only three gears – there are some hills we just won't be able to climb. For dealing with life-threatening illness, skills that many consider adequate are just not good enough, and both patients and clinicians are paying the price. To make matters worse, research shows that clinicians are unable to accurately evaluate their own communication skills. And even those who are aware of their shortcomings tell us they don't have confidence that they can change. In this book, we want to show you that change is possible, and you can become a better communicator. First, we describe what expert clinicians actually do when they talk to patients and their families. Second, we show what you can do to improve your practice. We highlight specific skills to emulate and offer suggestions for how to practice these behaviors. We want to raise the bar on communication skills. We want to change your idea of what really good communication looks like.

Where possible, we have grounded these recommendations in the growing literature on communication. Yet we've consciously distilled the communication tools and roadmaps into a reader-friendly format. This is not an academic review of the literature that stresses what we don't know. Our goal is practical – to help you communicate better.

How Is the Book Organized?

After discussing what it takes to become a better communicator (Chapter 1) and outlining foundational communication skills (Chapter 2), we organized the book in a progression that parallels how clinicians frequently work with seriously ill patients and follows them through their illness trajectory, including talking about serious news (Chapter 3), discussing prognosis (Chapter 4), planning for the future (Chapter 5), discussing in-the-moment treatment decisions (Chapter 6), managing life between the big events (Chapter 7), discussing goals of late-stage care (Chapter 8), conducting a family conference (Chapter 9), dealing with conflicts (Chapter 10), and talking about dying (Chapter 13). We've also included tips on talking with colleagues (Chapter 11) and what to do when you're really stuck (Chapter 12).

The last chapter (Chapter 14) will help you know what to expect as your skills improve, describes what getting better feels like, and offers advice on how to continue to cultivate your skills. In this revision, we have also introduced our awareness of the roles privilege, race, and power play in the medical encounter and offer some tools that we hope will help clinicians navigate this landscape with greater self-awareness and sensitivity. Throughout the text, we include snippets of real conversations, slightly disguised, from our own practice and from the courses we've taught. Our goal throughout is to provide you actual words to use.

Finally, we congratulate you for wanting to improve your skills. The first step in the journey is the hardest one. You have made that commitment by picking up this book.

Acknowledgments

This book rests on the shoulders of prior leaders in palliative care and clinician–patient communication. We want to particularly acknowledge Bernard Lo, Richard Frankel, Phyllis Butow, Susan Block, Mike Rabow, Timothy Quill, and David Weissman, from whom we have learned so much about communicating with seriously ill patients. Kelly Edwards had a crucial role in developing our pedagogy, and Walter Baile helped Bob, James, and Tony start VitalTalk.

The first edition of the book was written by Tony, Bob, and James. We feel blessed to have worked together for over 20 years in developing the book's core concepts. It has been a wonderful partnership in which the sum is better than the parts. Our countless discussions, while often heated, focused on the work and made our thinking better. We cannot imagine better collaborators and our shared effort has been a crown jewel of our academic lives. Having Elise, Gordon, and Holly join us in the second edition has brought both fresh ideas and delight at the work's generative power.

This book also benefits from the wisdom and collective experience of our VitalTalk family. These talented clinicians, who inspire awe as they bring their whole selves to this difficult work, have helped us refine our ideas and given us feedback about what works (and does not) in practice. Without the VitalTalk staff, no courses would have ever materialized, and we would never have been able to write this book. Their dedication and passion for the mission have made our jobs easier and their insights have continually improved our teaching. Special kudos go to Jennie Dulas and Lynsey Seabrook – previous and current VitalTalk leaders, and our very first staff persons – Jackie van Allen, Rose Schulte, and Lisa Barrett. We would like to thank Angie Jabine for her careful editorial review and Jessica Papworth at Cambridge University Press for her patience through many delays.

Writing books require the support of both one's work and personal families. Bob wishes to acknowledge Wishwa Kapoor, Alan Meisel, and Missy McNeil for their support and encouragement of his scholarly career. Colleagues in the Section of Palliative Care and Medical Ethics at the University of Pittsburgh, particularly Julie Childers, Rene Claxton, and Jane Schell, helped him refine his thinking on many of the concepts in the book and become a better clinician. Colleagues such as Doug White and Gretchen Schwarze helped him understand emotions, shared decision-making, and bioethics; Doug Lemov and the Masters of Science in Medical Education focused his learning on how to teach. Finally, his children, Brandon and Kirsten, dealt with his absences and distractibility and still became amazing adults.

Tony's deep gratitude flows to Diane Meier, Sean Morrison, Charles von Gunten, Kathy Foley, Roshi Joan Halifax, and J. Randall Curtis, with big appreciation to Anders Ericsson, Doug Lemov, Paulo Freire, and John Dewey. Much of the VitalTalk project's initial work was made possible by generous funding from the National Cancer Institute, the Arthur Vining Davis Foundations, the Gordon and Betty Moore Foundation, the John A. Hartford Foundation, and the Cambia Health Foundation. The Project on Death in America, part of the Open Society Institute, brought Bob, Tony, and James together. The Brocher Institute, outside Geneva, supported a writing sabbatical. Rock Health and the Impact Hub Seattle provided incubation support as a social startup. IDEO and the Stanford d.school provided training in design thinking. Jeannie Walla helped VitalTalk find its feet with actors, and The Gant in Aspen was for 20 years home base. Ted Gibbons patiently accompanied Tony through it all.

Elise is grateful to her whole VitalTalk family for the continuous cycle of mentorship, learning, collaboration, and friendship that makes the VitalTalk community what it is. Particular thanks go to the coauthors of this book, along with Kelly Edwards, Lynn O'Neill, Steve Berns, Jillian Gustin, Justin Sanders, Lynn Aliya, and Jennie Dulas. She also would like to thank mentors, friends, and colleagues who have influenced her path to and in this work – Mike Rabow, James Hallenbeck, Seth

Landefeld, Helen Chen, Steve Pantilat, Susan Block, Vicki Jackson, Rebecca Sudore, Kristen Schaeffer, Rachelle Bernacki, and Molly Feely. Finally, Elise sends gratitude and love to her fantastic family, Bill, Dan, and Gabe Carey, who tolerated years of travel with patience and love.

James grew up hearing his father's dinnertime stories about patients' lives and from them learned that sacred moments emerge when we listen deeply. He is grateful to both his parents for the values by which he strives to live. As a resident and fellow, he learned from too many young men with HIV/AIDS how to sit quietly with loss, and Bernie Lo and Margaret Chesney set him on the path to communication research. At Duke, he is grateful to Harvey Cohen for support and guidance, and to amazing research collaborators Kathryn Pollak and Karen Steinhauser, who gave interdisciplinary insight and methodological rigor, and made it all fun. For the past eight years, Dana-Farber Cancer Institute has offered an enormously generous and collegial environment in which to set his ideas into practice. Throughout, James' sons Noah and Zeke have kept him humble and laughing. And this book, as well as all that came before it, would never have happened without the love, encouragement, and nourishment from his wife Ilana Saraf.

Gordon is forever grateful to Stephen McPhee, Joshua Hauser, Michael Preodor, his coauthors, and all the VitalTalk faculty and staff for their friendship, mentorship, and partnership over the years. He would also like to thank Diane Wayne, Marianne Green, and the Department of Medical Education at Northwestern University for supporting this work. He would like to express special gratitude to his Northwestern teaching team, including Melanie Smith, Laurie Aluce, Eytan Szmuilowicz, and, in particular, Julia Vermylen, who codirects the program and has been an amazing partner since the very first course. Finally, none of this would be possible without the love and support of his wife, Czarina, and daughters, Eva and Penelope.

In addition to her coauthors and Kelly Edwards, who have indelibly changed who she is as a teacher and human, Holly wants to express her love and gratitude for Laurel Herbst, Charles von Gunten, Frank Ferris, Suzana Makowski, and Gary Buckholz. Among so many incredible people in the VitalTalk faculty and staff, Holly wants to specifically acknowledge Steve Berns, Wendy Anderson, and Michael Barnett for their care and helping her think more broadly about their work together, and Lisa Barrett and Ashley Look for their patience and partnership over the years. Special thanks are owed to the international faculty, especially the VitalTalk Down Under crew who have brought new joy and perspective to the teaching. Finally, Holly is grateful for the love and support of her family, especially her husband Joe Runnion.

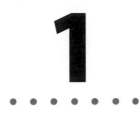

1

Taking Your Skills to the Next Level

The Challenge

Telling a mother of two that her colon cancer has returned – and it's incurable. Explaining to a schoolteacher with chronic lung disease that to continue working, he will need portable oxygen. Helping the parents of a five-year-old girl with metastatic neuroblastoma after treatment decide whether to enroll her in a clinical trial. Giving the news to an accountant with chronic hepatitis that her incidentally discovered hepatocellular cancer is unresectable, so she's off the transplant list.

These conversations are territory that many of us learned to navigate mostly by trial and error. Even after years of experience, we still take a deep breath before getting started and prepare for a discussion that will change the life of the person before us.

Patients and their families remember these conversations like they happened yesterday. They can recall exactly what was said, often word for word. They remember whether the clinician rose to the challenge with honesty, kindness, and resourcefulness or, rather, filled an awkward silence with medical jargon. They remember whether they left the visit hopeful, supported, or confused.

How clinicians handle these difficult conversations can make or break a therapeutic relationship. We've seen colleagues who take on the challenges and others who sidestep them. Most of those who steer clear of tough encounters have good intentions but don't know how to act on them. They worry they'll say the wrong thing, take away a patient's hope, cause a patient or family to break down or get angry, or open a Pandora's box that will take way too much time in a busy day. Or, they feel like no matter what they do, the patient (or family) doesn't hear them and gets upset anyway.

Compare those colleagues with expert clinicians who excel even during the toughest encounters. They seem to intuit what the patient needs. They know when to offer information, when to ask an open-ended question, and when to make an empathic comment. Rather than randomly "winging" it, they have a framework that guides their communication.

How do you talk with patients and their families about balancing hope with reality ... or trust with caution? Do you wish you were more confident about where to go with the conversation? Do you feel stuck when a patient asks, "Why me?" Do you get into arguments with angry family members? Do you find yourself unsuccessfully trying to convince some seriously ill patients that effective disease-directed therapies are no longer an option? And do you wish you had a more effective human response to patient suffering? If so, this book is for you.

Does Better Communication Really Make a Difference?

Let's be honest. Through the hidden curriculum, many of us were taught that if a patient gets the right tests and treatments, nothing else really matters. In medicine, attendings "pimped" us about the labs, the scans, or the treatments, and quality metrics focused on clinical outcomes – they didn't pay attention to whether we had explained the

diagnosis in a way that patients could understand. The implicit message was that communication is like the cherry on top of a sundae – a
nice touch but expendable.

We were misled. Research shows that communication is central to
the effective work of a clinician. Good communication improves a
patient's adjustment to illness, lessens pain and physical symptoms,
increases adherence to treatment, and results in higher satisfaction
with care. Poor communication skills are associated with increased
use of ineffectual treatments, lower adherence to therapy, and higher
rates of conflict. What's more, good communication doesn't just affect
patients; it also affects you. It helps you enjoy and thrive in your work.
Better communication skills are associated with less stress, less burnout, and even fewer malpractice claims. Suboptimal communication
creates a vicious spiral that makes us feel more like hamsters on a
wheel than like healers.

Clinical practice is changing in ways that put a premium on communication skills. Patients now have more access to medical information
than ever before, and they are avid consumers of this knowledge. They
Google their illness and raise questions about the most recent research
advances. As biomedical advances have made decision-making
much more complicated, patients and families need clinicians to add
the judgment and experience that they cannot get from a website.
Communication between patients and clinicians is more complex,
and has more layers, as clinicians must integrate a mountain of biomedical information with their patients' values, hopes, and priorities.
The Internet does not substitute for a skilled, caring clinician.

Finally, communication helps to build trust. Over the past 10 years,
the public's trust in professionals has decreased for a variety of reasons – sensationalized cases of bad actors, political polarization, the
rapid spread of misinformation, and the controversies around COVID.
Trust is particularly a problem among patients of color for whom a
long history of structural racism has led to inequities in care. Good
communication skills cannot fix these societal problems. However, the

data suggests that communication skills are associated with increased trust – a critical component of good care.

Can Clinicians Really Learn to Communicate?

When we lecture on this topic, one of the comments we hear most frequently is, "You can't teach communication. You pick up what you need from experience. Besides, some people are simply better at it than others." Well, it's true that some clinicians start out better than others. But communication is a skill that can be taught, and when it's not taught properly, the learning that occurs through trial and error is not always productive.

As clinicians progress in their careers, they don't see how others communicate – the interactions are usually private – and they only get feedback when they've been outstanding or have truly offended someone. So, most clinicians settle into communication routines. These habitual patterns are not necessarily bad, because they help us routinize our world.

However, the downside is that we may charge along in our work and overlook people's individual needs. The patient worries about quality of life and the clinician talks about survival. Or the patient wants information and the clinician keeps asking questions about coping. Either way, the routine leaves patients at least a bit frustrated and, worse, feeling isolated. Like the golfer who needs to correct their swing, clinicians need to consciously shed these bad habits. This can only be accomplished through learning new techniques and gaining experience using them. The good news is that sophisticated research shows that clinicians can indeed learn to communicate better. But not by doing the same old thing over and over. You need to see the medical encounter in a new way and observe differently what is happening. Then you can be more intentional about what you are trying to accomplish and more versatile with a wider array of communication tools. And, as a result, your patients will be more satisfied – and you will be too.

clinicians, even in the absence of well-tuned capacities, improve their communication skills. Patients respond! Even clunky expressions of empathy are usually well received. In the process, patients reveal more and draw their clinicians into a deeper and more authentic relationship which, in turn, hones their own capacities such as empathy and tolerance. In other words, good communication begets more good communication.

What Will Better Communication Do for You?

After our work was profiled in the *New York Times,* a physician wrote to describe his experience learning to communicate. As a young resident in the emergency room, he remembered asking his supervisor how to tell a parent that her child had died in a car accident. The attending physician's advice: "Don't let the family get between you and the door." It's a sad commentary on how clinicians learn and reminds us of the study in which oncologists cited "traumatic experiences" as the most influential source of learning communication.

Compare this to the feedback we received from one of our Oncotalk Fellows. He wrote:

> It remains clear that these conversations are difficult to have. Being surrounded by bad news does not necessarily make a person skilled at delivering it with compassion or clarity. Still, I listen to myself speaking to patients and using the tools I learned during my week in Colorado. I feel less flustered and my words are less tangled; I can focus on the person across from me and find out what is needed from me in that moment – and that seems like progress.

Even more enthusiastically, one oncology fellow sent us this email a week after completing a VitalTalk communication skills course:

> When I saw a patient today that was distressed, I was able to name the emotion, use empathic statements, and use praise statements. I never once used the word chemotherapy, death, dying, prognosis, or

treatment. The patient was able to get out what they needed and the conversation segued smoothly into moving forward from here and what we need to do to get there. As a matter of fact, he thought I was the best physician he had ever seen, and *I didn't even talk to him about his cancer*. I couldn't believe it. *It was freakin' amazing!* It was like a switch went off in my head, an epiphany, that if I just talk to patients in a way that provides alignment, I will be able to ultimately provide better care!

This seems like progress to us, too. Our measure of success for skilled clinicians is that they will be more capable of finding a way through a difficult conversation. We don't promise that the conversations will always feel simple or smooth or that better communication will enable you to escape sad situations. We can say, however, that many of the clinicians we train feel more engaged with their work, experience more connection to their patients, and get more joy from their practice. It's exhilarating to watch. We see clinicians who become more flexible and more resilient and develop a greater capacity for the work medicine requires.

What's Our Philosophy?

Over the past three decades, as people have sought to humanize the profession, we've watched waves of theory and nomenclature break over the practice of medicine. Terms such as "shared decision-making," "patient-centered," and "relationship-centered" have all been used in support of better communication. In this book, we are going to ignore the labels. For these situations, we think that the critical task for clinicians is to find a way to integrate complicated biomedical facts and realities with emotional, psychological, and social realities that are equally complex but not very well represented in the language of medicine. Working with life-threatening illness is a cross-cultural experience. As a clinician, you need to understand both the biomedicine and the personal story, and you need to be able to speak in both languages.

In these situations, communication is not about delivering an information pill and seeing how much the patient can swallow; it is about sending messages to the patient, receiving messages in return, and seeking to coordinate these in a way that leaves a patient informed and feeling heard and understood. This back-and-forth model of communication has some important implications. First, respecting the complete process of communication will lead to better outcomes. The preparatory steps we outline in the roadmaps may seem obvious to you – but for a patient who has never been in your clinic before, they can make a big difference. Second, communication is a two-way process. You must attend to what the patient is telling you. If you are too busy sending messages (e.g., giving information) to read the replies (e.g., hear the patient's emotional reaction), the conversation will no longer sync. It would be like talking to the patient while you are listening to their heart – you will likely miss the subtle murmur.

Our Basic Principles

Throughout this book, we will illustrate a few basic principles, but we've collected them here to give you the big picture upfront. These are more than pearls – they're the bedrock of our work.

1. Start with the patient's agenda. (Of course, you bring your own agenda; and first you must find out where the patient is coming from.)
2. Track both the emotional and the cognitive data you get from the patient. (Don't look past the emotion.)
3. Stay with the patient and move the conversation forward one step at a time. (Don't let yourself get ahead of the patient.)
4. Articulate empathy explicitly. (You are creating a safe conversational space.)
5. Talk about what you **can** do before you talk about what you **can't** do. (You need to show you are working for the patient.)
6. Start with big-picture goals before talking about specific medical interventions. (Ensure that you and the patient are aligned about what is most important **before** offering details about possible interventions.)

7. Spend at least a moment giving the patient your complete, undivided attention. (When patients tell you something big, put down your pen, stop typing on your computer, and show them you are listening.)

8. Ask your patients what they are taking away from the conversation. (This helps you evaluate how you are doing in the moment and what you can do to improve in the future.)

A Word about Emotion

In this book, we emphasize a distinction between "cognitive" and "emotion" data. Since both words have a variety of uses, we would like to clarify what we mean when we use them in this book. By "cognitive" data, we are referring to conscious intellectual processes like thinking, reasoning, and judging. When you're talking to Mrs. E about prognosis and she mentions that she read on the Internet that the five-year survival for her cancer was 50%, that is a piece of cognitive data. This particular piece of cognitive data tells us that she has consciously sought out information and tried to understand and comprehend it. Cognitive data tells us what patients understand rationally. On the other hand, when she flushes while she mentions this and you catch a look of distress flashing across her face, this is a piece of emotion data. Emotion is not under conscious control; it is involuntary. Mrs. E's flash of worry is a piece of emotion data that tells us this patient is having a tough time reporting what she has read because she is concerned about what it means for her. Emotion data tells us about a process of integration occurring in the parts of the brain that have to do with appraising value and creating meaning, because emotion processing prepares the brain and the rest of the body for action.

What does all this have to do with communication? In medical settings, we often hear clinicians frustrated, irritated, or overwhelmed with the emotion patients show, or we notice them trying to ignore emotion altogether. They dismiss emotion as human frailty and assume it has less value than cognition. In fact, emotion plays an important role: it determines how we decide what is valuable. And when you are talking to a patient with a life-threatening illness, figuring out what is truly valuable is often the most important underlying communication task. Besides, if this emotion is never acknowledged, the conversation will not move forward in a productive way. Responding to emotion is about much more than being nice; it's about being effective. We consider emotion data to be as important as cognitive data and will emphasize recognizing and responding to emotions.

Patients are not the only ones with emotions. Clinicians also respond in ways that can powerfully impact the conversation. The medical news causing the patient distress may also make you sad, as you contemplate losing a patient about whom you care deeply. Or, a patient's behavior may trigger you to feel annoyed or even angry. And, even more complicated, sometimes patients or their situations remind us of tender moments in our own lives. These emotions can create a veil through which we observe the clinical encounter. They may offer greater insight and empathy that enhances our therapeutic effect. Or, if not acknowledged and contained, they may interfere in our role as healers as we use the clinical encounter as a place to inappropriately process our own feelings. Our ability to use our own emotional data in the service of patients is a complex topic that falls under the realm of capacities discussed earlier and about which we encourage further study and, perhaps, personal work.

How to Use This Book

You can use this book in two ways. You can flip straight to the chapter that addresses a challenge you currently face. Each chapter contains a step-by-step guide, or cognitive roadmap, that will help you to find your way through a difficult conversation. Alternatively, you can read the book straight through. Read in order, the chapters are designed to build a set of skills that will build a repertoire of communication tools that is powerful and flexible.

Maximizing Your Learning

Athletes don't learn to put a ball in a basket or ski down a steep slope by reading a book. And musicians don't improve their tone and dexterity by watching a lecture. Skills, unlike medical facts, must be learned through observation, practice, and feedback. During VitalTalk courses, we demonstrate what good communication looks like so learners know what to emulate. We then teach using observed role-play – because the research shows that feedback is critical to putting new communication skills into practice. When learning on your own, consider ways that you can simulate this idea of practice with feedback. What follows are several ideas for you to enhance the skills we would teach at a course.

Record yourself. Listening to your own voice or watching yourself on a video is a humbling experience. (Do I really sound like *that*?) But it's worth the hassle (and the pain). Telehealth visits make doing this particularly easy. Don't forget to have your patient sign permission and make it clear that you are doing this to become a better clinician. Even cynical patients will be impressed that you are trying to improve. Listen for what you say and what you sound like when you're saying it. Better yet, have someone you trust watch or listen to the video or audio. Ask them to comment specifically on something you are working on.

Refine your observational skills. We've found that, prior to communication training, many clinicians do not consciously or sufficiently collect observational data – they are less skilled at recounting what happened. Lacking this observational data, they see communication as magical rather than a series of intentional decisions, words, or gestures. So, try to watch exactly what happens in your conversations. What did you say that worked? Or didn't?

Practice one new skill at a time. Communication is a complex psychomotor skill, and until you've mastered one thing, it's hard to focus on something else. You wouldn't try to learn to use your new mobile phone while driving a new car, would you? Pick **one** skill. And, the first time, pick something that doesn't feel too hard. Remember that the best learning happens in situations that offer a bit of a challenge yet aren't overwhelming.

Debrief yourself. After a difficult conversation, find a couple of blank sheets of paper and, for a few minutes, in private, write down everything you can remember about what happened. Include snippets of what you said and what the patient said, as well as reactions, emotions, body language, and the effect of the conversation on you personally. Don't censor anything, just get it all down on paper. We try to put our pen on the paper and just keep writing for two or three pages. If other thoughts intrude, just write them down, then get back to the conversation. Later, see if a lesson or an insight emerges.

Ask for feedback. Find someone else to watch you and give you feedback. If you work in an interdisciplinary team and round with other professionals, this can be the perfect setting. Keep in mind that many medical professionals do not have highly developed feedback skills: they ignore your goals, don't notice your strengths, and tend to say something nice just before they say something mean. Therefore, don't open yourself up to a known character assassin. Give the person something specific to watch for. Tell them you just want two or three observations relevant to a skill you are working on. Tell them you don't want their opinion about what you should have said – you want their observations (what happened?) about what you did say.

Be patient. Even though the authors of this book are supposed to be experts, we still find ourselves chagrined because we lack patience, feel insufficiently spiritual, distract ourselves with petty ambitions, and remain perplexed about some things. Anne Lamott said wisely that "perfectionism is the enemy," so remember that you just need to stay on the path. Your mistakes can be portals to new learning. And remember, if you are trying to improve in this realm, you've already distinguished yourself from most clinicians.

Pay attention to praise. Working with life-threatening illness has a long learning curve, but it has its rewards. When you get positive feedback, pay attention. Don't brush off a compliment ("It was nothing," "It's my job"). Breathe deeply, take it in, record what it was that you did successfully, enjoy the moment, and say "Thank you."

You're ready to begin.

Further Reading

Gottlieb, L., *Maybe You Should Talk to Someone*. Houghton Mifflin Harcourt, Boston, 2019.

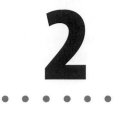

Foundational Communication Skills

Our goal in a VitalTalk workshop is that learners leave with at least one new communication skill to use the following week. Over the years, we have found four skills to be the most commonly named take-home points:

1. "Ask-tell-ask"
2. Recognize and respond to emotions
3. Ask permission to move the conversation forward
4. "Tell me more … "

In this chapter, we will describe these foundational skills and show how they serve as building blocks for all serious illness communication.

A Common Problem

All of us have left encounters wishing the conversation had gone better. As we've looked back at these challenging visits, we've realized that, more times than not, the conversation failed because it was missing one of the four foundational skills upon which we focus in this chapter.

Let's start with an encounter one of us (Gordon) had years ago with the sister of a 75-year-old woman with metastatic colorectal cancer. The patient had been admitted the night before with a bowel perforation. Initially she seemed stable, decided against surgery, and began conversations about wanting to go home with hospice. By the next morning she was delirious, tachycardic, and hypotensive. Gordon was called to see her in a new palliative care consultation and he contacted her sister who lived out of town. Below is the encounter in detail.

WHAT HAPPENED	WHAT WE CAN LEARN
Dr. W is rounding alone. The fellow is off for the day and frequent pages have left him running behind. After seeing the patient, he realizes that the team's prior plan for home hospice may not be possible given her declining mental status and unstable vital signs. He finds the number for the patient's sister and calls her to discuss changing the plan.	*The doctor is feeling harried and rushes into this conversation without considering how he plans to approach it.*
Dr. W: Hello, my name is Dr. Gordon Wood. I'm one of the Palliative Care doctors taking care of your sister. I'm sorry to hear everything you and your sister are going through this morning.	*Trying to build rapport, but assumes the sister is up-to-date.*
Ms. D: Umm … yeah … how's she doing?	
Dr. W: What have you been told?	*Recognizes he should "ask" before he "tells"*
Ms. D: I talked with her last night. I know she's pretty sick and she wants to go home with hospice.	
Dr. W: Yes, that's what the other doctors talked to me about as well. Unfortunately, seeing her this morning, she is starting to get confused and I'm worried that she may be declining quickly. I think we may need to reconsider whether she can go home.	*Mistaking her solemn demeanor as evidence of a good understanding of the very serious nature of her perforation, the doctor transitions to telling her that she is getting sicker and the disposition plan may need to be reconsidered.*

WHAT HAPPENED	WHAT WE CAN LEARN
Ms. D: Declining quickly? Can't go home? Are you saying she's dying? How can that be? I talked to her last night and she said everything was ok. I know she has cancer, but it doesn't grow that fast!	
Dr. W: I'm so sorry. It sounds like you may not have been told everything. Did she talk to you about the problem with her bowel?	*Realizing a gap in understanding the doctor needs to backtrack to ask again. He feels he needs to correct this misunderstanding. His focus on the information gap makes him also miss the patient's emotion.*
Ms. D: (escalating distress) She said she had some infection, but the antibiotics were working, and she was going home. She always tries to shield me from the bad stuff. What's going on with her bowel?	
Dr. W: Unfortunately, the problem is serious. The cancer has caused a hole to open in the wall of her bowel and despite antibiotics, I'm worried that she may die before she can get home.	*Now, with a realization of her true level of understanding, the doctor can start his "tell" of medical information at a more appropriate place. He gives a "headline" that describes what has happened and its meaning.*
Ms. D: Oh my god, that's awful!	*She has a better medical understanding, but the mishandling of the initial "tell" has escalated the emotions which have yet to be addressed.*

Although Gordon was trying to build rapport, assess the sister's understanding, and give news clearly, he didn't ask enough about her understanding to realize the gaps. This led to the unintentional disclosure of the patient's limited prognosis and resulted in confusion and unattended distress for the patient's sister.

The Problem: Patients, families, and clinicians often have very different understandings of the medical situation.

The Solution: Before "telling" new information, "ask" enough to ensure you are starting from the same place.

Ask-Tell-Ask

The conversation above would have gone differently if the doctor had used the first of the foundational communication skills discussed above: Ask-Tell-Ask. Ask-Tell-Ask is an approach to sharing serious news that underlies all the conversation roadmaps you will encounter in this book. It consists of three steps:

1. Ask what the patient (family) knows
2. Tell the "headline"
3. Ask what they understood

Using this approach to delivering serious news respects the patient or family by starting with their perspective. It also gives you a sense of what they already know, which tells you where to begin and how to frame the information. Finally, it helps you assess the effectiveness of your communication and allows you to clarify misunderstandings.

As simple as it sounds, Ask-Tell-Ask is a paradigm shift from what we often see. In many family meetings, clinicians typically start with a long summary of the medical information and then ask for questions. In some cases, patients clearly understand the situation and become frustrated by the long description of what they already know. Alternatively, a patient or family member's response may indicate a fundamentally different understanding of the medical context and the new information makes no sense, or even comes as a shock. In the example above, asking the patient's sister what she had been told by others could have avoided this problem. Finally, many patients and family come to us after already searching online for their own answers. Your not knowing what they have learned may lead to a situation where they judge you as knowing less than Dr. Google.

When first using Ask-Tell-Ask, a common mistake is to assume your work is done after one "Ask." Unfortunately, that first bit of information may be incomplete, as with Ms. D's description of her sister only as "sick" and wanting to go home with hospice. Gordon never asked, "Anything else?" or clarifying questions that would have revealed she did not fully appreciate the severity of the bowel perforation and the resulting shortened prognosis. Two, or even three, "Asks" are often needed to fully understand the patient or family member's perspective about the medical situation.

Asking what they know upfront serves other purposes as well. For example, asking "Have you done any of your own research on this condition?" helps you understand what the patient has learned from the Internet. If you are interested in what the family has been told about prognostic issues, you can ask "What have the doctors told you about what might happen in the future?" Before giving serious news, one might want to ask, "Is there anyone else who should be here when we talk?" or "Is this a good time to talk about what I know?" And, finally, since someone's trust in what we have to say may be influenced by prior experiences of prejudice, we've started to also ask the following question of new patients: "Have you had experiences with the medical team where you feel people treat you differently because of who you are?" Although we recognize that some may be uncomfortable with this question, we've found it to be extremely well received, lead to deeper and more authentic conversations, and help to establish our trustworthiness.

Our model for Telling is also different than what you may see in typical clinical encounters. The data suggests that when giving information, physicians provide long monologues that combine pathophysiology with extended explanations of clinical reasoning. Unfortunately, patients often don't understand the message because it's too technical for them (and they may be embarrassed to admit it). Moreover, the description does not answer the patient's core question – what does this mean for me? Our emphasis in Telling is therefore twofold: (1) the information should be at a sixth-grade level and (2) the message should be short and focused on what this means for the patient. (See "giving a headline" in Chapter 3.)

Finally, all communication is a leap of faith. We try hard to speak in a manner we think will be understood. However, despite our best efforts, we may miss the mark – our metaphors may be confusing or the concepts too complex. The only way to know this is to probe for (mis) understandings. This is the purpose of the second Ask which comes in two formulations. First, ask about patient questions. An ingenious study found that "What questions do you have?" is more likely to get a response than "Do you have any questions?" You may need to ask this more than once as patients frequently won't offer their "real question" initially, or need time to formulate what they really want to know. The second part of this "Ask" is the "Teach Back" question (www.teachbacktraining.org/). This identifies whether a patient heard what you were trying to say. To avoid shaming the patient, some clinicians preface the question with "I sometimes don't explain things as well as I'd like so I find it's important to check and make sure we're on the same page." A nice way to then truly ascertain what they've taken away is to ask, "Can you tell me, in your own words, what you're going to tell your family tonight about our visit?"

Ask-Tell-Ask: Beyond Delivering Serious News

As mentioned above, Ask-Tell-Ask is foundational to all the communication roadmaps presented in this book. It's useful to see how this approach can be helpful in even the most basic of communication tasks, such as setting an agenda for a visit. As an example, below is a roadmap for setting an agenda for a typical outpatient visit, that includes Ask-Tell-Ask.

1. *Make a welcoming statement.* Think of this as the beginning of the relationship – it should be inviting. If you are late, apologize. The apology

need not be long, but an acknowledgment of your lateness is important because it is common courtesy, and it establishes your commitment.

2. *"Ask"* *about the patient's main concerns for the visit.* Because patients often have more than one concern, it is often helpful to ask "Anything else?" to ensure you have all the patient's concerns before you get into the meat of the interview.

3. *"Tell"* *your agenda for the visit.* Clinicians usually have several things they want to make sure are covered. Articulate these for the patient.

4. *Propose an agenda for the visit* that meets that patient's concerns and your concerns. This agenda is the beginning of your shared goals for care.

5. *"Ask"* *the patient for feedback about the agenda.* Does your proposal seem like a reasonable plan to the patient? If not, the goals for the visit may need to be revisited.

Let's look at an example of an encounter Tony had where he used the above roadmap to set an agenda.

WHAT HAPPENED	WHAT WE CAN LEARN
Dr. B: Hi, are you Mrs. Stevens? I'm Doctor Tony Back, you can call me Tony. I apologize for being late today, but I'm all yours now.	*Acknowledging lateness.*
Mrs. Stevens: Hi, you can call me Ann.	
Dr. B: I got a note from your surgeon, Dr. H, that you were here to talk about breast cancer, yes?	*Volunteering information that shows continuity with the referring doctor.*
Ms. A: nods.	
Dr. B: What are the big issues that you want to make sure I cover today?	***Asking*** *explicitly about the patient's concerns.*
Ms. A: I want to know about the best treatment and the options for my stage of cancer.	
Dr. B: We will definitely cover that. Anything else?	*Setting the agenda with "anything else?"*

WHAT HAPPENED	WHAT WE CAN LEARN
Ms. A: I'm also very concerned about my quality of life during treatment. Those are the main things for today.	
Dr. B: Great, because those are two of the things I wanted to cover also. Just so you know, I like to hear about your concerns at the beginning of our visits so I can be sure that we talk about them. In the future you can bring a list of questions if that works for you.	*Beginning the negotiation of the shared agenda by **telling** the doctor's concerns and setting an expectation for agenda-setting in future visits.*
Ms. A: I'd appreciate that. Thank you.	
Dr. B: You're welcome. So, for today, here's what I propose. I'll spend a few minutes going over your history, to make sure I've got it straight. Then I'll do a brief exam. Then we'll use most of the time to go through those two big issues – the treatment options, and how this affects your quality of life. How does that sound to you?	*Making a proposal for a shared agenda and **asking** for the patient's assent.*
Ms. A: Sounds fine.	

Recognize and Respond to Emotions

The second foundational communication skill we will discuss is the ability to recognize and respond to emotions. When we encounter difficult situations in our practices, this is probably the skill that we most often use to navigate toward a solution.

Why It's Important to Recognize and Respond to Emotions

Emotion interferes with cognition. It's useful to imagine that patients experience clinical encounters through an emotional channel and a cognitive channel. And they typically process through one channel at a time. For example, when a clinician discloses a cancer diagnosis, patients often receive this in the emotional channel which overwhelms their ability to incorporate new cognitive information about the treatment plan. In fact, this has been demonstrated in functional magnetic resonance imaging (fMRI) studies that show how emotional experiences light up the limbic system in the brain and shut down the cortical cognitive centers. This explains why patients say, "I didn't hear anything after the word 'cancer.'" Recognizing this phenomenon helps us understand why sharing information in that state is not only unkind, it's ineffective. If you can respond to the emotions until they lessen, patients have the space to move to the cognitive channel at their own pace, and you can discuss further medical information at a moment when the patient can hear it. Even when that transition occurs, emotions may continue to bubble up and we hear from patients that they want their clinician to be responsive and to toggle between the emotion and cognitive channels as needed.

Emotion should not, however, be thought of as merely an impediment to cognition. Recognizing and responding to emotion is helpful for other reasons. First, it builds connection. Studies show that attending to emotions is correlated with both patient satisfaction and trust. Second, emotions provide data that hint at what is important to the patient. For example, if a patient responds to a new cancer diagnosis with tearful concerns about how her husband with dementia will fare if she is sick, you need to respond to that emotion before discussing the treatment plans. The emotional response tells you how important her husband is to her and that you need to incorporate the care of her husband into the plan you discuss.

Why Clinicians Don't Pay More Attention to Emotion

There are a variety of theories about this, but we think that most clinicians just haven't learned how to deal with emotion in the context of a medical visit. We hear clinicians say that they feel pressed by time, worry about opening a "Pandora's box," and feel uncomfortable with strong emotions.

The core of empathy is the ability to identify and appreciate another person's emotional state. Neurobiologists have discovered "mirror" neurons that enable us to place ourselves metaphorically into the shoes of another person. For a clinician, the skill is to use that mirroring capacity and not become completely absorbed in it. Thus, one must possess the capacity to "create a place to hold the patient," from which one can shuttle back and forth – feeling their emotion and your emotion. Without this skill, the emotion can seem like way too much to deal with. How do you get there? You must build your awareness of your own emotions and your ability to tolerate your own strong emotions. This will allow you to be present, and even therapeutic, in the presence of your patient's strong emotions. If you can do this, the data also suggests that visits in which emotions are attended to are actually shorter than those where they are not. In other words, we don't have time NOT to attend to emotion.

How to Recognize Emotions

Verbal displays of emotion are often obvious. Patients may angrily ask for who is at fault or sob as they lament losing a lifelong partner. Sometimes, however, emotions may present in more subtle ways. For example, repeated questions that keep coming, even when thorough answers have been given, is a common way for emotions to mask as a "cognitive" response.

Nonverbal displays of emotion are ubiquitous. We all respond to each other nonverbally – with facial expressions, hand gestures, body positions, and objects (think about glancing at a watch). While most of the communication research in medical encounters has focused on words, nonverbal communication could be even more important. People tend to exert less conscious control over their nonverbal gestures, and thus nonverbals may be more telling – important to remember when you are facing a patient who is sitting stiffly with crossed arms and lips pressed into a thin line. However, nonverbal communication is also less specific and is easier to misinterpret. The task is to think of a patient's nonverbal and verbal displays of emotions as a kind of clinical data, similar to how patients' telling their illness story serves as data about their understanding of their medical situation.

How to Respond to Emotions

Learning to respond to emotions in an explicit way may seem silly – after all, aren't we all responding to people's emotions constantly? But the conscious use of emotional data is a skill that you will need to hone to optimize your ability to communicate.

The way we respond is a process called empathy. Empathy means putting yourself in the other person's shoes and imagining what his or her life is like. Put simply, empathy means "I am trying to imagine what it would be like to be you." Empathy is not just a nice intention; real empathy shows up on brain scans as a specific kind of function. Responding to emotion, though, requires empathy and then action. To be therapeutic, it's not enough to recognize what the patient is experiencing – you must convey your understanding to that patient. Many clinicians entered health care because they wanted to utilize this capacity, but the process of training can leave us a little bit numbed, and even feeling that the capacity for empathy can be a liability.

Understanding emotion data and how you can respond can help you cultivate empathic capacity, and in our experience, the sense of liability gives way over time to something much richer.

A *simple framework* for recognizing and responding to emotions looks like this:

1. Commit to observing and using emotional data in your communication.
2. Notice the patient's emotion, and name it for yourself.

3. Refrain from trying to fix or quiet the patient's emotion – this may require that you pay attention to your own worries and not act on them immediately.

4. Acknowledge the emotion explicitly. This can take many forms. Nonverbal responses may include silence, eye contact, changing position, or perhaps touch. Verbal responses may be expressions of understanding, support, and respect, or exploration when you know something is going on but are uncertain of what it is. The acronym N-U-R-S-E summarizes the most common and effective verbal responses to emotion (see box "Responding to Emotions with Words").

RESPONDING TO EMOTIONS WITH WORDS

Patient's emotional statement: "These headaches are killing me!"

Clinician's empathic responses:

N	NAME the emotion:	"It sounds like this has been frustrating."
U	UNDERSTAND the emotion:	"It must be so hard to be in pain like that."
R	RESPECT (praise) the patient:	"I'm impressed that you've been able to keep up with your treatment and the rest of your life while having these headaches."
S	SUPPORT the patient:	"I will be here with my team to help you with the headaches."
E	EXPLORE the emotion:	"Tell me more about how these headaches are affecting you."

Fischer, G., J. Tulsky, and R. Arnold, Communicating a poor prognosis. In: R. Portenoy and E. Bruera, eds., *Topics in Palliative Care*. Oxford University Press, New York, 2000.

The clinician's capacity to acknowledge and talk about emotions requires some care in word choice. In general, you will do better to understate the patient's emotion and to show curiosity: not "You look furious" but "I'm wondering if you're concerned." Patients may feel labeled when they are recipients of unskilled "emotion naming." Many already have the impression that "good patients" don't emote too much and calling it out too strongly can magnify that sense.

As you learn to recognize and respond to emotions, we encourage you to be as specific as possible. Distress, frustration, sadness, and melancholy differ from each other, and the more accurately and nuanced our acknowledgment of emotions, the more successfully we convey our empathy. This requires practice (much like one learns to identify the different tastes in wine by tasting a lot of wine!). The good news is that if you try to name an emotion and get it wrong, the patient will often correct you, both building your relationship and helping you be better next time.

Motivational Interviewing (MI) offers another way to acknowledge emotions. Reflective listening is the most central MI skill and can also be the most challenging to learn. There are two types of reflective responses: (1) **Simple reflections** essentially repeat back to a patient the exact content of what he or she has said; (2) **Complex reflections** include the patient's unspoken meaning, feelings, intentions, or experiences. Complex reflections are a way to guess the emotions behind a patient's words. ("It sounds like given all you have done to try to get better, it's frustrating to hear that your heart is getting worse.") Complex reflections are a highly effective way of responding to the patient's emotions, naming motivations that are implicit in the conversation.

Another effective tool to respond to emotions is the "wish statement." For example, if a patient desperately says, "There must be another treatment you can offer!" you can respond with, "I wish there were more treatments that would help." We find this particularly powerful because it demonstrates partnership – we want the same thing as the patient (i.e., an effective treatment), while implicitly confirming that this outcome is not possible. Notice that when using the wish statement, there is no need to complete the second half of the sentence ("... but there aren't any"). This is understood, and leaving it out emphasizes the alignment rather than the bad news.

Whichever words you choose to respond to a patient's emotions, the task is usually one of finding a toolbox of phrases that feel natural to you. What works for one person may not work for others and the only way to find what works for you is with practice.

Asking Permission Before Moving a Conversation Forward

The third foundational communication skill we discuss here is: Asking permission before moving the conversation forward. In this book you will see lots of conversation maps for tasks like discussing serious news or clarifying goals of care. When clinicians start using these maps, they often get stuck in how to transition between steps. Asking permission to transition to a different topic is an incredibly effective skill that helps you decide whether the patient is ready for the next step on the map. For example, we often see trainees who work hard to develop skills at recognizing and responding to emotions but then do not know how to transition the conversation from feelings to discussing the medical decisions at hand. It is often a turning point in their development as communicators when they can notice the moment that emotions have calmed and can ask permission to move forward. It sounds something like this: "Thank you for sharing that with me. It's very helpful. Do you think you're ready to talk a little about what comes next?" In the upcoming chapter, you will see another common application of asking permission that helps the transition between understanding what the patient has heard ("Ask") to informing them of serious news ("Tell").

While asking permission is quite effective, we find that it may seem, at first, unintuitive. Aren't we leading the conversation? Isn't permission implied? What if they say no? Don't I still need to tell them? These are all questions we hear frequently. We find asking permission so helpful because it gives patients and families some control in a situation that often feels very out of control. It also serves as a signpost that clearly identifies a transition in the conversation which is helpful to both patients and clinicians. We also find it provides useful information about their readiness to proceed. You may think someone has calmed down, but when your request to discuss the treatment plan is met with sobbing, you know they need some more time before they can hear what you want to discuss. Recognizing the power of this tool, one of us (James) has observed that the greatest change in his communication style over the past 15–20 years is likely how often he asks permission.

Two final points. First, in response to asking permission, anything other than a strong "Yes" should cause you to pause. Given your social power, answers such as "I guess" or "If we have to" should lead to an inquiry before proceeding. Naming the ambivalence ("It sounds like you're unsure whether that's something you're ready to talk about") or asking for more information ("Tell me more") will help you decide on the next steps.

Second, if the patient says "No," it means you cannot raise the new topic without further discussion. Nothing is more disrespectful than asking if it is okay to talk further and then ignoring the answer. Rather than talking about the topic, you can talk about the issues surrounding the topic. Imagine a patient saying, "I don't really want to talk about my prognosis." It might help to notice the emotion driving this state-ment. ("It sounds like talking about the future is scary.") Alternatively, the patient might be willing to talk about their reasoning. ("Help me understand your view.") Finally, the patient might be willing to discuss the positive and negatives in talking about the future. ("Can you tell me more about not talking about the future?" or "Can you imagine a time when it would be helpful for us to talk about prognosis?")

Although prognosis discussions can usually be delayed, an emergent treatment decision may make that challenging. In these cases, nam-ing the urgency can be helpful. ("I know this is a difficult topic and I worry that there are some urgent decisions we need to make.") When a patient or family still do not want to be a part of that discussion, iden-tifying someone else to help with decisions can be useful. ("I know this is a lot. Sometimes patients ask that I talk to a family member. Would it be okay if I talked with your son?")

"Tell Me More"

We often find ourselves lost in a conversation. Things may have gotten a bit off track, the patient has dropped an unclear hint about what's on their mind, or we just don't really understand what the patient is trying to say. At those times, we've found that using the simple phrase "tell me more" can be an incredibly powerful tool. It demonstrates curiosity, maintains one in relationship with the patient while you're trying to figure things out, and may enable the missing details to be uncovered.

There are several different ways you might use this phrase. First, you may be in a situation where you think a patient has a straightforward informational need, but you're not sure what that is. Asking directly, "Could you tell me more about what information you need at this point?" might help clarify. For example:

> PT: "I'm having so much trouble deciding whether I can manage at home after I leave the hospital."
> CLINICIAN: "Could you tell me more about what information might be helpful at this point?"
> PT: "Honestly, I need to know how much it would cost to hire a nursing aide, at least for part of the time. If I could afford that, it would make all the difference."

The second, and perhaps most effective, use of this tool is after a patient has shared a bit of information that doesn't really explain what they're thinking but suggests they might be willing to go forward. For example:

> PT: "I'm just wondering about it all."
> CLINICIAN: "Tell me more … "
> PT: "Well, I don't really know how much time I have, and I need to know that if I'm going to make any plans."

In this case, "wondering" could have meant a lot of things, but "Tell me more" elicited the key information that this patient is wondering about prognosis, which will guide the conversation in a very specific direction.

Finally, this skill can serve as a gentle way to probe deeper into a patient's experience and elicit thoughts that might not bubble up otherwise. For example:

> PT: "I've just not been able to get my life back together since the diagnosis."
> CLINICIAN: "Could you tell me more about what this means for you?"
> PT: "Well, I feel like I'm living on borrowed time, and I have no idea what to do with that. But, I guess I'm mostly worried about the burden I'm creating for my husband and kids."

Virtual Communication

In 2023, we'd be remiss not to acknowledge that telehealth has changed the practice landscape, and some clinicians are conducting 75% or more of their visits virtually, usually over a platform like Zoom. "Webside manner" differs from its face-to-face counterpart, and the unique challenges force us to make even better use of our foundational skills. A few key points are worth considering. First, although the patient sitting in their living room may feel more comfortable than in the sterile clinic environment, they may also not be in the proper "head space" to see their clinician. They may have just disciplined a child, hopped off a pressured work meeting, or cleaned dog poop off the rug. This creates more need for the clinician to set the context for the visit, particularly if one expects to discuss weighty topics. Second, because we lose many of our nonverbal cues, verbal expressions of empathy become even more important. For example, silence or intensive eye contact, which can feel caring in the office setting, may appear strange over a screen and the gaps more awkward. If you feel the need to use some sort of nonverbal expression, some have suggested placing a hand over the heart to convey empathy. Third, because sometimes the natural flow of a conversation is interrupted, particularly with wireless bandwidth challenges, one must be slower and more deliberate in moving a conversation forward, and asking permission becomes even more important.

A Common Problem, Reconsidered

Now that we've discussed the four foundational skills (Ask-Tell-Ask, Recognize and Respond to Emotion, Asking Permission before Moving a Conversation Forward, and "Tell Me More") let's reconsider the case of Ms. D who has colorectal cancer and presented with a perforated bowel and how it might have gone differently using these skills.

WHAT HAPPENED	WHAT WE CAN LEARN
Dr. W. is rounding alone and getting frequent pages but takes a moment to call the primary team to clarify their communication with the patient's sister (none) and think about how he wants to proceed with the conversation.	*In the midst of a busy day, a moment of preparation and getting on the same page with all involved parties is invaluable.*
Dr. W: Hello, my name is Dr. Gordon Wood. I'm one of the Palliative Care doctors and your sister's doctors asked me to see her. Did anyone mention I would be calling?	*Knowing that only the ER and not the primary team had called him, the doctor starts at the beginning by asking if she even knew that he'd be calling.*
Ms. D: I talked to my sister last night and she mentioned that someone would be calling to help us get her home with hospice. I know she's pretty sick with this cancer and she told me that's what she wants. (sounding sad)	
Dr. W: I can imagine it's hard to be far away when she's this sick.	*Recognizing and responding to emotion.*
Ms. D: It is. Thank you for your help.	
Dr. W: Did she talk about what brought her into the hospital this time?	*Asking what she understands about the situation at hand.*
Ms. D: She said she had an infection, but everything was okay with the antibiotics, and she just wanted to go home.	

WHAT HAPPENED	WHAT WE CAN LEARN
Dr. W: Have you received any updates about how she's doing today?	*Asking if she knows about the clinical change that occurred that morning.*
Ms. D: No, but when I called her just now, she was confused, and it has me worried.	
Dr. W: Tell me more about that …	*Exploring further to assess a full sense of her understanding.*
Ms. D: Well, I've never seen her like that before and I'm wondering if she's changing more quickly than I thought.	
Dr. W: That's scary to think about. Is it okay if I tell you a bit more about what brought her in and how things have changed overnight?	*Acknowledges the emotion and asks permission to transition from the ask to the tell.*
Ms. D: Please.	
Dr. W: Unfortunately, the infection is pretty serious. It was caused by the cancer which created a hole in her bowel. I worry that the antibiotics are no longer working, and that's why she's getting more confused.	*Now, with an understanding of what she knows about what he needs to tell her, he can fill in the gaps and frame it appropriately.*
Ms. D: I was worried there might be more to the story, she always tries to protect me (getting tearful).	
Dr. W: I can tell how much you both care about each other.	*Recognizing the emotion and responding with a respect statement.*
Ms. D. Through thick and thin we've always had each other's backs (calmer).	*While still emotional, she has heard the information and is becoming more reflective.*
Dr. W: Would it be okay if we talk about what this means in terms of her wish to go home?	*Asking permission to transition to talking about a management plan. Here he is set up to discuss this in a much better way than the first time.*

The Bottom Line

The four foundational skills described in this chapter help you reframe communication from giving an information pill to sending and receiving messages about both emotional and cognitive data.

Maximizing Your Learning:

1. Commit to asking before telling with one patient in the next week.
2. After the visit, debrief yourself about what happened. How did you frame your ask? How did the patient respond? Did it have any effect on the rest of the visit?
3. Give yourself a reminder to try again. Try a sticky note, or a line on your to-do list. And remember to debrief. You need repetition to incorporate and become confident about a new skill.

Further Reading

Back, A. L. and R. M. Arnold, "Yes it's sad, but what should I do?" Moving from empathy to action in discussing goals of care. *J Pall Med*, 2014, **17**(2):141–4.

Chua, I. S., V. Jackson, and M. Kamdar, Webside manner during the COVID-19 pandemic: Maintaining human connection during virtual visits. *J Pall Med*, 2020, **23**(11):1507–9.

Coulehan, J. L., F. W. Platt, B. Egener, et al., "Let me see if I have this right … ": Words that help build empathy. *Ann Intern Med*, 2001, **135**(3): 221–7.

Epstein, R. M., Mindful practice. *JAMA*, 1999, **282**(9): 833–9.

Graugaard, P. K., K. Holgersen, H. Eide, et al., Changes in physician–patient communication from initial to return visits: A prospective study in a haematology outpatient clinic. *Patient Educ Couns*, 2005, **57**(1): 22–9.

Jacobsen, J., V. Jackson, J. Greer, and J. Temel, *What's in the Syringe? Principles of Early Integrated Palliative Care*. Oxford University Press, 2021.

Kripalani, S. and B. D. Weiss, Teaching about health literacy and clear communication. *J Gen Intern Med*, 2006, **21**(8): 888–90.

Kruser J. M., K. E. Pecanac, K. J. Brasel, et al., "And I think that we can fix it": Mental models used in high-risk surgical decision-making. *Ann Surg*, 2015, **261**(4): 678–84.

Levinson, W., R. Gorawara-Bhat, and J. Lamb, A study of patient clues and physician responses in primary care and surgical settings. *JAMA*, 2000, **284**(8): 1021–27.

Miller, W. R. and S. Rollnick, *Motivational Interviewing: Helping People Change* (3rd ed.). Guilford Press, New York, 2013.

Quill, T. E., R. M. Arnold, and F. Platt, "I wish things were different": Expressing wishes in response to loss, futility, and unrealistic hopes." *Ann Intern Med*, 2001, **135**(7): 551–5.

Silverman, J., S. M. Kurtz, and J. Draper, *Skills for Communicating with Patients*. Radcliffe Medical Press, Oxford, 2005.

Stone, D., B. Patton, and S. Heen, *Difficult Conversations: How to Discuss What Matters Most*. Penguin Books, New York, 2010.

Suchman, A. L., K. Markasis, H. B. Beckman, et al., A model of empathic communication in the medical interview. *JAMA*, 1997, **277**(8): 678–82.

Talking about Serious News
When the Emotional Channel Is On High

A new diagnosis of a serious, potentially life-limiting illness is a turning point for patients and clinicians alike. For patients, a diagnosis signals entry into what one writer called "the country of illness" – a complex world involving loss, decisions, therapies, waiting, and work. For clinicians, the capability to make these diagnoses and the responsibility that follows is powerful. Telling patients about a life-limiting illness raises complex emotions – sadness, powerlessness, and fear. If you've had a long-term relationship with the patient, having to share news that you know is life-altering is profoundly sad. Serious news may also cause us to reflect on the limitation of medicine's power and to feel impotent when we cannot alter a bad outcome. Finally, as the bearers of serious news, clinicians may worry about patients' reactions – will they blame us or be angry?

Serious news does not encompass only the initial diagnosis of a cancer or the repeat bad scan. It's learning you have diabetes, that now you must start insulin, or that the next treatment will have some bad side effects. It can even be as simple as "We were not able to draw your blood" or "The doctor is going to be 45 minutes late." Thus, what the medical literature has called "breaking bad news" has become a fundamental task in the communication repertoire.

We have renamed this task from "breaking bad news" to "talking about serious news." After years of teaching "how to break bad news," we became concerned that framing the task this way tacitly encourages a view of this skill as information dumping. "Talking about serious news" frames the task more constructively for the clinician and the patient. We're not backing away from the sadness or badness of having a serious illness, but we are orienting the clinician to the task at hand. The goal of the clinician faced with delivering serious news should be more about helping patients to understand diagnoses and come to terms with their new reality than about forcing them to confront brokenness. Patients have told us that rather than labelling the news as good or bad, they'd prefer we share information, and they can decide about what it means for them.

Skating on the Surface of the Emotion Data

Let's start by considering a case. In the excerpt below, Mr. Clark, a man treated for non-Hodgkin's lymphoma a year earlier, is in the office to learn the results of a computed tomography (CT) scan ordered in response to a lactate dehydrogenase (LDH) rise.

WHAT HAPPENED	WHAT WE CAN LEARN
Dr. B: Mr. Clark, how are you?	
Mr. C: Oh, I'm good, thanks.	
Dr. B: Okay, let's talk about what your lab tests and CT scan showed.	*Didn't check in to see what the patient is worried about or what he knows.*
Mr. C: I'm ready, I guess.	
Dr. B: On your labs, the LDH has gone up a little bit more.	*Starting to give the news. Trying to forecast news that lymphoma has recurred with the news about the LDH. Ignored the hesitation in "I guess."*

WHAT HAPPENED	WHAT WE CAN LEARN
Mr. C: Hmm, okay.	*The patient does not seem to understand that the doctor is giving bad news.*
Dr. B: On the CT scan, there are some enlarged lymph nodes in the chest. And in the abdomen. It's a surprise –	*Using the "enlarged lymph nodes" to disclose cancer recurrence – doesn't use the word "cancer." And is this a good surprise or a bad surprise?*
Mr. C: Yeah?	*Again, the patient does not seem to "get" that the news is serious.*
Dr. B: – certainly not what we were expecting. I know you've been feeling so well.	
Mr. C: Could we back up a little?	
Dr. B. Sure.	
Mr. C: So, you say the lymph nodes are back? Does that mean the cancer is back?	*Patient tries to clarify.*
Dr. B: Yes.	
Mr. C: So, everything I went through, it's going to start all over again. Is that what you mean? I'm back at square one, basically?	*The patient finally understands the news and predictably responds with emotion. This comment reflects distress as the patient questions whether his previous suffering from the cancer treatment was worthwhile. There is also some anger here.*
Dr. B: In some respects, yes; in some respects, no. I would like to talk a little more about this, is that okay?	*Trying to keep things "rational" rather than "emotional."*
Mr. C: I don't know what to think right now. I just went through so much to get back to normal. And I've tried to be so much healthier, to take care of myself so much more. (pause) To know that it's back, is hard for me to understand. I mean, is there any doubt?	*Patient is still reacting to the news.*

WHAT HAPPENED	WHAT WE CAN LEARN
Dr. B: Well, I feel pretty confident that this is what it is. It's the return of the lymphoma. I know you had a tough time before, but I want you to know that this is still treatable.	*Responding to the cognitive issue without responding to the emotion. Trying to reassure the patient prematurely.*
Mr. C: Treatable? Like it was treatable last time?	*Patient doesn't sound reassured.*

In this excerpt, the doctor has been completely accurate and truthful about the medical issues, and even respectful about when to move forward. But by backing into the news by discussing labs and CT findings, he leaves the patient confused. In the end, it's the patient who has to ask if the cancer is back. Once the news is clear, the patient's distress is palpable, and the doctor hasn't acknowledged it. The doctor tries instead to reassure but doesn't know exactly what the patient is distressed about. The result is reassurance failure because the reassurance is premature – Mr. Clark doesn't think the doctor understands him. No wonder clinicians can become cynical about their ability to help patients who are distraught. Given the nature of the news, there is no way Mr. Clark is going to leave the doctor's office feeling happy. However, if this physician had talked about the news clearly and noticed and responded to the emotion data as well as the cognitive data, the patient might have left feeling cared for rather than feeling he had to struggle to understand.

Pitfalls when giving serious news: Conveying the news vaguely or with jargon and overlooking the emotional data.

The Solution: Give a clear "headline," track the emotional data, and respond to it.

A Cognitive Map for Talking about Serious News

The map we use is "GUIDE" (Get ready, Understand, Inform, Demonstrate empathy, Equip your patient for the next steps). While similar to a popular map developed by Robert Buckman and Walter

Baile called "SPIKES" (Setting, Perception, Invitation, Knowledge, Emotion, Summarize), we prefer GUIDE because the name avoids the violent metaphor, and describes the clinician's goal when talking with patients about serious news. Here we describe the steps to emphasize the process of communication.

1. ***Get ready*** *before sitting down with your patient.* Ask yourself: who, what, when, where, why, and how.
   - *Who should be there?* Think about both the clinician and family side. Is there a chaplain or nurse with whom the family has grown close? Can the visit be timed so the spouse can be present? If the family can't be physically present can they join by videoconference or phone? Should the conversation be recorded for them?
   - *What is the news I want to share?* The clearer you are about the diagnosis, prognosis, and treatment options, the better the conversation will go. It is also important, prior to the conversation, to get all involved providers on the same page. In the hospital, a premeeting where everyone agrees on the message to be shared is critical. For early learners, we suggest even writing this down to decrease one's cognitive load during the conversation.
   - *When should we have this conversation?* Set a time when you can devote your full attention and that also works for the patient/family.
   - *Where should we have this conversation?* Find a reasonably quiet place in which you can all sit down. Have tissues in the room and pagers on silent mode. If talking to the family of an incapacitated patient in the hospital, ask if they want to meet in the patient's room or elsewhere.
   - *Why this conversation – what is its purpose?* Are you just conveying the information or is there an urgent decision that also needs to be made?
   - *How will I have this conversation?* What is my headline – what words do I want to use? If there are multiple providers in the conversation, who will discuss what?
2. ***Understand*** *what the patient has heard before you disclose.* Starting the conversation by asking what a patient understands or expects can provide an important window into the patient's perspective, especially if you are meeting the patient for the first time (remember Ask-Tell-Ask). If you ask, "What have you heard from the clinicians so far?" and the patient replies,

"No one has told me anything," you need to do some preparatory work before giving the news. The patient may in fact have been told very little, or more likely, the patient did not fully understand previous explanations. On the other hand, if the patient replies, "I have a three-centimeter spiculated mass in my right lung," this indicates that the clinician should be prepared to meet the patient with information at a more technical level. After understanding what the patient has heard, use our foundational skill of *asking permission* to transition to the next step in which you will disclose the news. Asking permission can seem superfluous – isn't it obvious that the patient is here to talk about the news? But think of this as a way to allow the patient to shape how the serious news is discussed. Simply asking patients, "Are you ready to talk about this?" gives them a bit of control and establishes that you want to work cooperatively. When you are working with patients from cultures that may have different expectations around the sharing of serious news, it may also be useful to ask, "Some people like to hear the medical information themselves, while others would prefer we talk to their family. What would be best for you?"

3. **Inform**, *or disclose, the news using a "Headline."* In journalism one can tell a story in two ways: start broad and narrow to a conclusion or start with the conclusion and expand with the details. Most stories start with the headline because it's easier for the reader. The other approach is generally reserved for long-form articles that assume a patient audience. In medicine, it's akin to ripping off a band-aid quickly versus slowly removing it and spreading out the pain. The data suggests that most patients prefer to have it ripped off quickly. When sharing serious news, we recommend applying this principle by starting with the "headline." You may need to eventually give more details – to better explain the situation, respond to patient and family questions, and demonstrate your knowledge and trustworthiness. However, this can wait until after the primary message has sunk in.

   If prior to giving the news you suspect that it will come as a complete surprise, consider prefacing your headline with a warning statement. (We don't like the metaphor of "firing a warning shot.") A few preparatory words can allow patients to brace themselves for negative news. For example, "The blood tests for your kidney function came back and there is some serious news we need to discuss."

The headline itself consists of two parts – what is wrong, and what does it mean. It should be jargon-free and end with the core information in plain language. The first part might look like, "Your dad came into the hospital because he had an infection. Despite all of our treatments, he's getting worse, and his lungs, kidneys, and brain are failing." The second part needs to focus on what this means for the patient's life – either in terms of longevity or quality. We often introduce this with language such as "I'm worried … " or "This means … ." In this case, you might say, "I'm worried that your father will not survive this illness." When there is a lot of new information with significant ramifications, you may need to break the news into smaller chunks. This can all appear easy on paper, but the more enculturated you are in the world of medicine, the harder it is to describe reality in simple language. Until this becomes second nature, you may consider even writing out headlines before delivering them.

Sometimes, the news is unclear or there are a range of possible outcomes. In these cases, one can say "It's hard to know at this point how he will do," and to remember that uncertainty is serious news as the listener is likely to worry that things will not go well. Another option is to use "hope and worry" language. For example, after a stroke, a clinician could say "While I hope your mom recovers most of the ability to use her left arm and leg, I worry she may not."

Finally, be careful about mentioning future treatments in your headline. This is a natural thing for clinicians to want to do because it makes the "bad news" seem less bad. And if the illness is curable, the meaning of the diagnosis is less severe. An oncologist may say, "The biopsy showed a Hodgkin's lymphoma which, with treatment, is curable." However, the treatment itself is serious news and many patients may progress despite therapy. In another example, even if dialysis or transplantation is an option, kidney failure is still life-altering.

In some conversations, sharing serious news is the prelude to talking about what should be done next (see Chapter 8, Goals of Care in Late-Stage Disease). If you say "Your lungs are getting worse and I worry that if this continues you will need to go on a breathing machine," you are prejudging what should be done. If a patient is told they "need" to go on a breathing machine, doesn't it mean that's the correct choice? In such a case, it might be better to say, "Your lungs are getting worse and I worry that we are going to need to make some really difficult decisions about what to do next."

Finally, after you give your headline, **be silent** and let the patient or family take the information in and respond before you say more. Immediately after hearing the headline, many patients feel numb, or their minds are racing in a swirl of thoughts and emotions. It is not quiet for them, and further information from the clinician can feel like an assault.

4. **Demonstrate empathy**. If you have given a clear headline, you will likely notice a wave of emotion that follows the news, and this wave will probably not subside until long after the visit is over. The clinician's job is to recognize and respond to the emotions (see Chapter 2). You need to notice the emotion, give it some space, and incorporate it as an influence in the discussion that follows. NURSE statements, as described in the previous chapter, can be very helpful here. To be sure, acknowledging the emotion won't make it go away. But responding to the patient's fear, anger, or numbness can provide a human dimension to a technical medical discussion and demonstrate that you care for the whole person.

You should continue to respond to patients' emotions until they have calmed down enough to hear cognitive information about what is next. Patients may tell you they are ready when they ask "Okay, what comes next?" Other times, you may have to check in by asking, "Is it okay if I move forward to talk about the plan and the options?" Watch the patient's response carefully. If he or she responds to this with more emotion, continue to respond empathically rather than moving forward with cognitive information.

5. **Equip your patient for the next steps in care**. At the end of the visit, be sure to summarize what you've discussed and describe concretely the next steps the patient will need to take. Although the patient may still be in an emotional state that does not allow them to fully grasp details, you want them to leave with as complete an understanding as possible. Here, we return to the second part of Ask-Tell-Ask and inquire "What questions do you have?" as well as request a "Teach Back" (see Chapter 2). A brief written outline done during the visit can be extremely helpful to a patient and family later and save your time in the future by reducing confusion.

Let's rewind back to Mr. Clark and see what happens when the doctor uses these steps and tracks the emotion more explicitly:

WHAT HAPPENED	WHAT WE CAN LEARN
Dr. B reviews the CT scan and notes recurrent cancer. He considers prognosis and treatment options before entering the room.	*Getting ready before he sits down with the patient.*
Dr. B: Nice to see you. How are you feeling today?	*Greeting the patient and checking on urgent issues.*
Mr. C: I'm doing okay. The pain meds have helped, and I got that CT you wanted.	
Dr. B: What did you understand about why we got that CT?	*Understanding what the patient knows.*
Mr. C: That lab test was high, so I think we were seeing if that meant the cancer is back.	
Dr. B: Is it okay if we discuss the results?	*Asking permission to transition to the news.*
Mr. C: (nods).	
Dr. B: Unfortunately, the scan shows the cancer has come back in your chest and belly.	*Informing the patient of the news using a one-sentence "headline."*
Mr. C: Oh, my god.	
Dr. B: (takes deep breath, waits).	*Using silence to give the patient time to respond. Silence works when the doctor provides an "empathic space" by sitting near the patient, possibly putting his hand on the patient's shoulder, and keeping the focus on the patient – not writing or typing.*
Mr. C: How can this happen?	*Emotion: shock.*
Dr. B: It's a shock to me, too. I was hoping not to see cancer.	*Demonstrating empathy by naming own emotion, echoes patient hopes.*

WHAT HAPPENED	WHAT WE CAN LEARN
Mr. C: But I've been so healthy. I gave up red meat. I did all that chemo before. That was supposed to help. Should I have gotten more?	*Patient still shocked, searching for explanation, starting to move into disappointment.*
Dr. B: You did everything right, everything possible to prevent this. I'm very disappointed too.	*Naming disappointment and praising the patient for his efforts in fighting the cancer.*
Mr. C: How will I tell my kids?	
Dr. B: We'll work with you on that. It's hard to talk to your kids and it's very important.	*Responding to worry by offering support to help the patient manage this challenge, and underscoring the importance of the patient's concern.*
Mr. C: Okay, what about the treatment?	
Dr. B: We can definitely talk about that if you think you're ready.	*Checking in to make sure the patient is emotionally ready to discuss next steps.*
Mr. C: (deep breath) Yes, what can we do?	
Dr. B: Let's start by discussing the treatment options.	*Equipping the patient for the next steps in care.*

The emotional subtext in this conversation is much more evident than in the previous one. The patient's concerns are more obvious, more in your face, more raw. His distress is right on the surface and, at first blush, this conversation looks like it would be more difficult. Yet the reality is that, for a clinician who can deal with the emotions, this conversation is actually easier because you know more about the patient's reaction. When you know what the concerns are, you can address them more directly. The result is less time spent on issues you assume will be worrisome that actually are not, and more time spent on the issues that count.

What If the Family Says, "Don't Tell"?

One special situation worth discussing is when a family member asks you not to tell the patient about their diagnosis. What makes this difficult is that in some cultures, patients expect (and want) their family to be told the diagnosis rather than them. A beautiful film, *The Farewell*, illustrates this well (www.npr.org/2019/07/24/744805282/filmmaker-lulu-wang-based-the-farewell-on-her-family-s-real-life-lie). Knowing how to how to respond to this request is thus an important cultural competency for providers who disclose serious news. Nondisclosure raises ethical questions about which all parties have strong conflicting opinions. In such cases, if patients are told their diagnosis, then families feel ignored and disrespected. Yet not telling a patient may violate her autonomy and your conscience. The conflict can often be avoided by using the previously discussed skills of asking before telling and attending to emotions empathically.

Start by attempting to understand the family's point of view. Remember: in virtually all cases, the family has the best interests of the patient at heart. "Tell me about your concerns" is a much better way to start than "We have to tell her." It's open-ended and will help show the family that you are interested in their story. You may find out that the patient had clearly stated that he or she did not want to be informed of bad news and preferred to defer to family members. In other cases, families assume patients' views based on how similar situations were handled in the past. Where family members presume patient agreement with nondisclosure, the clinician may suggest the possibility that the patient might have a different opinion. "I wonder how we would know if your mother did want to know more about her illness?"

In most cases, however, families base their desire to "protect their loved one" from bad news on a belief that the news will cause unnecessary suffering. They want to protect their loved one from feeling the distress that they are feeling. It is therefore important to respond empathically to families' emotions. An example of such a response might be, "I understand this must be a difficult time for you and your family." Or "I see how worried you are." (Interestingly, these behaviors may help the family feel more confident that you will talk to their loved one in a sensitive way.) In discussing the family's view, it is important to respectfully talk about the implications of not telling the patient the diagnosis, for example, "I wonder if you have thought about some of the practical issues associated with not telling your mother about her diagnosis. Can I mention some of my concerns?" For example, if a request is made to inform a patient with cancer that he or she has an infection, families generally have not considered how to explain the necessity of treatment in a clinic with a sign that includes the word "cancer."

In our view, the challenge is to figure out what the patient wants to know, without disclosing the news in the process. The simplest way to do this is by asking patients directly how much information they want to hear. This is best done early in the course of an illness, although we are not always afforded this luxury. In discussing this with the family, it is important to be explicit that the goal is *not* to talk the patient into doing this one way or the other. "I'm fine with you (the family member) being the decision maker, if that is what she wants. I just want to confirm that, so we are doing what she wants."

As a part of this negotiation, certain ground rules and possible outcomes should be considered in advance. First, role play with the family about exactly what you are going to say to reassure them that you are trying to be respectful to the patient's wishes. We tell the family that we are going to say to the patient "Some patients want to be told directly about their illnesses and others would prefer for the family (or a specific individual) to be in charge. What do you want in this regard?" Second, you should talk with the family to identify who will share information with the patient if it turns out the patient does want all the information. Finally, you should discuss if the family wants to be present for this conversation with the patient or whether they want you to do it alone.

LISTENING BETWEEN THE LINES

I was seeing an Asian woman with metastatic pancreatic cancer. The primary team asked me to talk to her about her diagnosis and its implications. I went in to talk about the CT done the previous day and "give her the bad news." But before I even gave her the news, the patient volunteered that she had been caring for her daughter's father-in-law. She was incredulous that the "doctors had told him his diagnosis" – of cancer. When I asked what she meant, she said, "Doctors should never tell patients that they have cancer, they should talk to their family. It is too much of a burden to tell a patient." She was telling me that she did not want to know her own diagnosis. And she reminded me how important it is to ask permission before giving serious news.

The Impact of Technology on Talking about Serious News

The rapid advance of technology has only made the clinician's job in discussing serious news harder. Information flows rapidly through the electronic medical record and patient portals so patients may discover information before we even see it. This is yet another reason why it is so important to check a patient's understanding before disclosing information. However, setting expectations in advance may be an even better way to navigate these challenges. For example, in oncology clinics, visits are often prescheduled shortly after planned scans to discuss results. A clinician could say,

> We're meeting on Thursday to go over your scan from Tuesday. Some patients find it hard to avoid reading the report on the medical portal before we have a chance to talk. Can I explain why I think that is a bad idea? I worry that when people read the report they see a lot of words that need a clinician's interpretation. If you read it before we talk, it may cause confusion and unnecessary worry. Therefore, I often ask patients if they can wait and we can go over it together.

Patients are also more used to asynchronous communication over email or text and may press for more information before a visit. If patients or families press for information over email or the phone, you can discuss why you think it is better to talk in person. You may say, "I appreciate how important it is for you to hear the news quickly. And I also want to make sure I've had a chance to learn everything I need to know, and that when we talk I can be sure you hear the full context." If pushed, a telephone call can at least allow you to use the steps of GUIDE and help navigate the emotions associated with the news, although the loss of ability to see nonverbal behaviors make it more challenging. Before disclosing serious news over the phone, make sure they are in a safe place and ideally have someone to support them. Of course, a virtual video visit is now another common option that overcomes many, but not all, of these challenges.

If the News Is a Medical Error

Medical errors are not the main focus of this book, but it is worth mentioning the importance of such disclosures. The roadmap is very similar to what we've described earlier as the error is serious news. What needs to be added to the headline is an apology.

An apology has three parts. First, it must acknowledge that the health care team made an error. ("We made a mistake.") Second, clinicians should express remorse over the error rather than explaining or excusing the error. The simplest way to show remorse is to say "I'm sorry." The apology is stronger if it acknowledges the consequences of the action on the patient. ("I know this means you will be in the hospital longer and I regret that.")

Finally, the data suggests that patients and families want to know what will be done to prevent similar errors from occurring in the future. Equipping the patient to trust the health care system requires your explaining what is going to be done to prevent the error in the future.

When patients find out about errors in a roundabout way, and don't receive a direct explanation, they lose trust in the health care system. The apology is an attempt to repair trust. The possibility of maintaining some trust lies in your willingness to come clean and offer the apology. What most clinicians will need to deal with before they offer the apology, however, is their own guilt, and this is part of the preparation for this particular type of serious news.

The Bottom Line

When giving serious news, start by understanding what the patient knows, give a clear headline, and try to be responsive to both the patient's cognitive AND emotional needs.

Maximizing your Learning

1. Give yourself a few minutes to think back to a memorable incident in which you were giving serious news. One way to do this is to write in a journal the first things that come to mind. Don't worry about grammar, penmanship, or coherence. Don't judge anything as good or bad, just pay attention to what comes to mind. Sometimes even writing is too exclusively left brain, so if you feel constrained by writing, just sit back (in a quiet place) and open your mind to images, feelings, sensations. Just collect them and see what comes up. How have these stories or images or feelings influenced how you approach giving serious news?

2. Choose one new skill from this chapter to work on – just one! We want you to focus your learning energy. For example, if you want to practice making empathic comments, choose a starting place, such as, "I'm going to acknowledge sadness when it comes up." Then commit yourself to trying it in clinic – tomorrow or next week. Make yourself a reminder, and a time to debrief yourself (this could be as simple as the time on your drive home).

Further Reading

Back, A. L., S. B. Trinidad, E. K. Hopley, et al., What patients value when oncologists give news of cancer recurrence: Commentary on specific moments in audio-recorded conversations. *Oncologist*, 2011, **16**(3): 342–50.

Baile, W. F., R. Buckman, R. Lenzi, et al., SPIKES: A six-step protocol for delivering bad news: Application to the patient with cancer. *Oncologist*, 2000, **5**(4): 302–11.

Barclay, J. S., L. J. Blackhall, and J. A. Tulsky, Communication strategies and cultural issues in the delivery of bad news. *J Palliat Med*, 2007, **10**(4): 958–77.

Childers J. W., A. L. Back, J. A. Tulsky, and R. M. Arnold, REMAP: A framework for goals of care conversations. *Oncol Pract*, 2017, **13**(10): e844–e850.

Delbanco, T. and S. K. Bell, Guilty, afraid, and alone: Struggling with medical error. *N Engl J Med*, 2007, **357**(17): 1682–3.

Eggly, S., L. Penner, T. L. Albrecht et al., Discussing bad news in the outpatient oncology clinic: Rethinking current communication guidelines. *J Clin Oncol*, 2006, **24**(4): 716–19.

Friedrichsen, M. J., P. M. Strang, and M. E. Carlsson, Breaking bad news in the transition from curative to palliative cancer care: Patient's view of the doctor giving the information. *Support Care Cancer*, 2000, **8**(6): 472–8.

Manning, A. and N. Amare, Bad news first: How optimal directness depends on what is negated. 2017 IEEE International Professional Communication Conference (ProComm), 2017: 1–10.

Parker, P. A., W. F. Baile, C. de Moor, R. Lenzi, A. P. Kudelka, and L. Cohen, Breaking bad news about cancer: Patients' preferences for communication. *J Clin Oncol*, 2001, **19**(7): 2049–56.

Porensky E. K. and B. D. Carpenter, Breaking bad news: Effects of forecasting diagnosis and framing prognosis. *Patient Educ Couns*, 2016, **99**(1): 68–76.

Ptacek, J. T., E. A. Fries, T. L. Eberhardt, and J. J. Ptacek, Breaking bad news to patients: Physicians' perceptions of the process. *Support Care Cancer*, 1999, **7**(3): 113–20.

Truog R. D., D. M. Browning, J. A. Johnson, and T. H. Gallagher, *Talking with Patients and Families about Medical Error: A Guide for Education and Practice*. The Risk Management Foundation of the Harvard Medical Institutions, Inc., 2011.

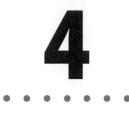

Discussing Prognosis
A Tightrope Walk between Hope and Reality

When discussing prognosis, clinicians face a series of contradictory impulses. For many, telling patients that their illness will take their life, particularly when they include a time estimate, makes them feel like they are giving a "death sentence." It's easier to let these issues slip away and focus visits on symptoms, logistics, and treatment options. On the other hand, these same clinicians know that when patients don't realize how close to death they really are, they often fail to make plans and miss a key opportunity to achieve life closure. They may also delay expressing goals for care, leaving families and clinicians to make decisions for them – often with conflict and heartache. Thus, for many clinicians, the impulses to both inform the patient and avoid a discouraging discussion coexist.

Patients have their own contradictory impulses. Surveys consistently reveal that patients want a great deal of prognostic information. For example, in one British study, 87% of patients wanted "all possible information." Yet patients also warn clinicians about being "too blunt," and say that "supporting hope" is very important. To further complicate matters, a significant minority of patients want to avoid prognostic information altogether, and in some cultures talking about a poor prognosis risks creating a self-fulfilling prophecy. How can clinicians possibly get this right?

Finally, both patients and clinicians must deal with the limitations of data. Survival statistics, such as mean and median, address the average outcome for a population. However, individual patients follow their own trajectories, and some will be the outliers on the survival curve. Many patients who hear the data and fully understand the implications of a 5% five-year survival rate are also fully convinced that they will be one of that lucky 5%. Clinicians share this optimistic bias. A study that asked physicians to predict survival for their patients being referred to hospice found that they offered more optimistic prognoses the longer they had known the patient. Why? Perhaps because it is difficult for clinicians to foretell death for patients to whom they are emotionally attached.

Realists, Optimists, and Avoiders

Given these conflicting motivations, it's no surprise that clinician behavior is quite variable. We find that the majority fall into three groups, which we call "realists," "optimists," and "avoiders." These strategies correlate with research that shows that 37% of physicians would tell a patient an accurate prognosis, 40% would be partially accurate (and usually optimistic), and 23% would decline to discuss prognosis altogether, even if asked directly. Each strategy is based on a core principle – and each also comes with unintended consequences. Realists emphasize that they support patient autonomy; patients need to understand their situation accurately to make good decisions. The unintended consequence is that realists can come off as blunt and even brutal. Optimists emphasize that they support patient hopes; patients look to clinicians for encouragement and a sense of what's possible. The unintended consequence is that optimists sometimes leave patients and their families unprepared for dying. Finally, avoid-ers emphasize the limits of statistical information and the inability to predict an individual disease course; patients don't benefit by receiving inconclusive data. The unintended consequence is that avoiders can seem cold, evasive, and unwilling to share their expertise and experience, thus leaving patients struggling to make sense of their prognosis.

Clinicians and patients influence each other in how much discussion of prognosis occurs. One extreme version of this mutual influence was depicted in a study that showed physicians and patients tacitly agreeing to a "Don't ask, don't tell" arrangement or colluding to avoid discussing the uncomfortable facts about disease. The patients generally learned about their prognosis by talking to other patients in the waiting room who were further along in the illness, or they discerned it from their own bodily decline. And therein lies the crux of the matter: patients navigating serious illness have thought about the possibility of dying, and they think about their prognosis whether we discuss it with them explicitly or not. When we bring it up, we aren't giving them the idea; we are merely giving them an avenue to discuss what is already on their minds, hopefully in a way that keeps them better informed and helps them feel supported.

> **The Pitfall:** Assuming you know what the patient wants to know about their prognosis.
>
> **The Answer :** Ask patients how they want to talk about prognosis.

The Prognostic Awareness Pendulum

Prognostic awareness is neither singular nor stagnant. Gary Rodin and colleagues have written about the phenomenon they call "double awareness," which refers to the "capacity of individuals with advanced cancer to sustain and negotiate the dialectical tension that arises between remaining engaged in the world, while preparing for impending death." In other words, people living with a terminal illness can hold both things simultaneously – an understanding that death is near, and an ability to banish those thoughts, so that they can live their lives. Juliet Jacobsen and colleagues have described this as a pendulum swinging between moments of worry or understanding and moments of hope and optimism. Over time, and even within one conversation, patients may express both perspectives. For clinicians this can be mystifying and even exasperating. You've had a clear conversation with the patient, thought you were on the same page about prognosis, and then you hear the patient say something unrealistic and inconsistent with your recent discussion. Know that this is normal!

But, if your patient is bouncing back and forth between these two poles, how do you respond? Well, in addition to the specific communication tips described in detail below, it's probably less about what you say and more about how you say it. Appreciate the emotional context behind these swings, remain nonjudgmental and don't seek to correct the patient. Patients' vacillating responses are data about how they are processing their illness, and by allowing them to express their hopes and worries, you can build a deeper connection.

Negotiating What to Talk About

Because many patients want some prognostic information and because there are so many types of prognoses to talk about (disease-free survival, overall survival, likelihood of surviving a year, response to a treatment, anticipated functional status, or cognitive decline, etc.), it's difficult, if not impossible, to predict what a particular patient wants to know. Whereas we know that a patient's educational level correlates with a desire for more information and more advanced illness correlates with wanting less information, such general trends are not useful when faced with an individual patient. A clinician can only give the "right" amount of information after understanding what the patient wants to know, and patients report that they want to negotiate when and how to talk about certain topics. Therefore, we recommend a negotiation-based strategy for dealing with prognosis.

The Opening Question: How Much Do You Want to Know?

We find that patients can generally tell us what they want to talk about and with what level of detail. Thus, we start with a simple opening question: "How much do you want to know about what the future may bring?" The question has a couple of functions. It invites a response that goes beyond "yes" or "no," and it establishes prognosis as a topic where a certain amount of give and take between clinician and patient is possible. If the patient struggles with this question, the clinician might help normalize a range of possibilities by saying, "Some people want lots of details, some want to focus on the big picture, and some would rather not discuss it at all. What would work best for you?" How the patient responds informs the clinician as to how best to navigate the conversation going forward. We find that patients most commonly give one of three types of responses: they want explicit prognostic information; they don't want any prognostic information; or they are ambivalent about receiving prognostic information, meaning that they both want and don't want it simultaneously. Ambivalence may be the most common response.

Discussing Prognosis with a Negotiation-Based Approach

We'll describe how to discuss prognosis in each of these three situations (they want to know; they don't want to know; or they're ambivalent), as well as offer some general pearls. However, regardless of how you choose to approach the discussion with the patient in front of you, make sure you know all the essential information about that patient's prognosis *prior* to initiating the discussion. This includes what might happen with different treatments and their responses. It's also helpful to confirm your assessment of prognosis with the patient's other providers – perhaps the primary care physician (PCP) or cardiologist – before talking to the patient. This allows you not only to check your own understanding but also to take a collaborative approach to the patient's care. This demonstrates to the patient that the various members of the medical team are working together on their behalf, and it also proactively engages other providers as potential additional sources of information and support for the patient and family.

Keep in mind that, as mentioned earlier, a patient's understanding of their illness and prognosis evolves over time, as their illness progresses and their function changes and as they work to cope with living (and ultimately dying) with a serious illness. As such, these conversations are not one-offs – they are iterative, and they need to evolve along with the patient's understanding, coping, willingness to talk, and decision-making needs.

A Roadmap for Talking about Prognosis with Patients Who Want the Information: ADAPT

Just like other forms of serious news, discussions about prognosis can be life altering. Therefore, you'll notice the similarities between ADAPT and GUIDE for talking about serious news. Yet prognosis differs from other types of serious news in that patients are often ambivalent about discussing it, may view this information as optional, or may simply disagree with our sense of what the future might bring. As you enter the discussion, be guided by a recognition that patients are more likely to understand and retain information they desire to hear.

1. ***Ask*** *what they already know about the future of their illness.* This will give you a sense of the patient's current understanding as well as what new information they might need. You might say something like, "What have the other doctors told you about what to expect with this illness?" or "What's your understanding about what the future may hold?" The kind of answer they give (e.g., optimistic, pessimistic, realistic, or uncertain) will direct how the rest of the conversation flows and allow you to correct any misconceptions. If they respond dismissively with something like,

"No one can predict what will happen," you might respond with a broadening statement like, "Of course, I can't predict exactly. If it would be helpful, what I can do is give you information about the best case, the worst case, and what's most likely."

2. ***Discover*** *what information your patient wants and negotiate the content of the discussion.* Clinicians can negotiate information sharing by establishing a patient's information needs and proposing ways to meet those needs. These negotiations enable patients to indicate their interest and readiness to hear specific types of information. For example, in response to a patient who says, "I want to know my prognosis," the clinician might say, "What kind of information about the future would help you plan?" If the patient seems stuck, the clinician could say, "There are several ways I can answer your question, so tell me which would be best for you. One way I can answer is to give you some statistics – the average time a person with this disease at this stage lives. Or, sometimes people have a specific event in the future they are wondering about, and whether it's realistic to reach it. Which one of these would you find most helpful?"

3. ***Anticipate ambivalence*** *when you ask how much they want to know.* You can't talk people out of ambivalence or "solve" it with persuasion. What you can do is borrow a tool from motivational interviewing, name the ambivalence and invite them to articulate the pros and cons. You might say something like, "Most people want to know about their prognosis and don't want to know at the same time. How about you?" If they seem receptive, this can be followed by, "What do you think could be helpful about talking about prognosis?" And, "Is there anything you're worried might happen if we discuss this topic?" This groundwork may seem time-consuming, but the investment may pay off in your ability to help a patient absorb information they need and, with ambivalence, want.

4. ***Provide information*** *about what to expect in the future.* At this point, you should know if your patient is interested in hearing prognostic information and what type of information they want. With the context set, a clinician can share even difficult information about poor prognoses straightforwardly. If a patient has said, "I want to hear the average length of time that a person with this disease lives," then the clinician can answer, "The studies for patients with metastatic colon cancer show that half of the patients have died by two and a half years, and about 95% have died by five years." One sentence, such

as this, is enough before you should stop, pause, and check in. Give facts slowly, in small, bite-sized chunks, to allow the patient time to digest and react to the data before you continue. This is like the "headline" concept you read about in Chapter 3 – you want to give a brief overview of the essential information concisely and clearly, linking the facts to their meaning. This is tough information to share, and it is even tougher to hear. As such, we find it helpful to think through (and maybe even practice) the words you will use to discuss prognosis with the patient before you enter the room.

5. ***Track emotion,*** *and respond with empathy, acknowledging the patient's and family's reaction to the news explicitly.* The patient and family are likely to have an emotional response to prognostic information, particularly if it is serious news. We commonly observe clinicians withdraw from these emotional reactions, although our experience is that verbal acknowledgment of the reaction can facilitate a deepening of the conversation. For example, you may say, "It looks like that information was not what you were expecting," or "I can see this is upsetting." For this step, we recommend empathic statements that demonstrate explicitly that the clinician perceives the emotion, respects the emotion, supports the patient, and/or wishes to understand the patient's situation and explore their response. (See "Responding to Emotions with Words" in Chapter 3 for a list of empathic statements that can be helpful.) While empathic silence can be extremely powerful, in this particular situation, silence alone can leave patients unsure whether they can talk to their clinician about their emotional reactions.

A sample conversation with a patient interested in information and its follow-up is shown here:

WHAT HAPPENED	WHAT WE CAN LEARN
Dr. T: We've been talking a lot about where you are with your illness. Would it be helpful for us to talk about the prognosis for this kind of cancer and, perhaps, what kind of information might be useful?	*Asking the opening question.*
Mr. K: I need to know how long I'm likely to live. I have plans.	*He is a patient who wants explicit information.*

WHAT HAPPENED	WHAT WE CAN LEARN
Dr. T: If you don't mind telling me a bit about your plans, I might be able to give you information that is more useful.	*Negotiating the content of the discussion.*
Mr. K: We have a trip planned with my oldest friend and his wife in the fall, and my granddaughter is graduating in the spring.	*This is his personal context for the information.*
Dr. T: Okay, that's helpful. So, I think it's very likely that you will be able to go on your trip, since that's coming up in a few months. I even think that you have a reasonable chance of making your granddaughter's graduation a few months after that.	*Providing information in the context of the patient's personal timetable.*
Mr. K: (silent)	*It is useful to try to imagine, "What is he thinking?"*
Dr. T: Is that what you were expecting?	*Acknowledging the patient's reaction by empathic exploration.*
Mr. K: I'm just relieved, I guess.	
Dr. T: I know that talking about prognosis can be … well, touchy.	*Making another empathic response.*
Mr. K: You're right about that.	
Dr. T: Do you want to discuss more today?	
Mr. K: Not really. But I probably will another time.	*This was important. Knowing that the patient wanted information, the doctor might have been tempted to share more specific survival data. However, as he learns here, that would not have been welcome. He has already met the patient's need.*
Dr. T: So, can you share with me what you're going to tell your wife about this conversation?	*Checking for understanding.*
Mr. K: That you said that I would probably make it to our granddaughter's graduation.	*The patient has understood accurately, if with a somewhat more optimistic bias.*

WHAT HAPPENED	WHAT WE CAN LEARN
Dr. T: And we can discuss more next time. Do you think she might want to be here for that?	

These conversations unfold over time, so the following encounter picks up at a subsequent visit.

WHAT HAPPENED	WHAT WE CAN LEARN
Mr. K: I've been thinking – we talked about my granddaughter's graduation, but, really, what kind of time are we talking about? Years?	*Now, after processing some of the information, he appears to want more detailed statistics.*
Dr. T: Is that something you want to talk about? Do you want to hear about how long patients with stage 4 colon cancer typically live?	*Negotiating the content of the discussion.*
Mr. K: Well, I suppose so. But can anyone really say?	
Dr. T: I don't know how long an individual person will live. What I can do is tell you the average for a group of people living with this kind of cancer.	*Setting up the ensuing discussion for the patient to appreciate the difference between population and individual estimates.*
Mr. K: Okay. I'm a planner so I want to know the facts.	*He sounds very clear about the benefits for him.*
Dr. T: So even though I'm not able to predict exactly how long you will live, here's what I can say: Most people with metastatic colon cancer who have cancer in the liver and are getting anticancer treatment live for months to years. What I mean by this is that in a worse-case scenario, people live for a few months, and in the best-case scenario, they can live a few years. If you look at the average for all patients with this kind of cancer, it's about two years. Because you are otherwise pretty healthy and have responded well so far to all the treatments, I am hopeful you will do better than most. Does that make sense to you?	*Providing the information.*

WHAT HAPPENED	WHAT WE CAN LEARN
Mr. K: Yes. Well, I guess that's kind of a relief.	*Hmm. I'm not sure what his reaction means, so I'll check.*
Dr. T: Tell me more about what you mean?	*Acknowledging the patient's reaction by empathic exploration.*
Mr. K: I thought it was going to be worse than that. I had a friend who had this and only lived a few months. Although two years isn't really that good, is it?	
Dr. T: I wish it were longer. This is just an average figure, though, and not a prediction for you personally. I'm hoping you will do better. You are healthier than a lot of patients I see with cancer and that's a good sign.	*Acknowledging the patient's reaction.*
Mr. K: Thank you for being so clear.	
Dr. T: You're welcome. Just to make sure I explained things well, could you tell me what you're taking away from our conversation today?	*Checking patient understanding.*
Mr. K: That I'm healthier than some other people with this cancer and maybe I can do better than average, which is about two years.	
Dr. T: I think you've got a very good understanding of the situation. Now let's move on …	

For Patients Who Don't Want Information

Some patients will indicate in response to the opening question that they do not want to discuss prognostic information, leaving the clinician in an awkward place: on the one hand, wanting to respect the patient's wishes, yet, on the other hand, worried that hopes rather than facts may cloud patient decision-making. Four general principles are useful in these situations. First, remember that emotions (e.g., sadness and fear) often underlie motivations not to talk about the future. Attending to these emotions will build your relationship and may make it safer to talk about difficult things. Second, understanding why a patient doesn't want to know may – paradoxically – enable a clinician to find a way to discuss a difficult subject. Third, decision making does not always require that the patient understand detailed prognostic information. Confronting patients with information they don't want can be a waste of time, and even actively counterproductive. Patients may feel "browbeaten" with the truth or that the clinician is not "on their side." Finally, although some patients may not want to talk about prognosis, they may be more than willing to let you share this information with a surrogate. A trusted loved one can help ensure that the patient's decisions are based in reality (or can step in for the patient when necessary).

1. *Try to elicit and understand why the patient doesn't want to know.* Although we observe many clinicians simply backing off after hearing that a patient does not want to talk about prognosis, we find that understanding the patient's view can provide insight into their reasoning and coping. In fact, the discussion about why someone doesn't want to talk can be a useful trust-building step. For example, a clinician could initiate this discussion by saying, "I wonder if it might be helpful to talk about some of your worries related to this discussion?" Or, "If you could help me understand your thinking about why you would rather not talk about prognosis, it will help me know more about how to discuss other serious issues." A patient might reveal that he is sad and worried that discussion will deepen his sorrow, or that he is concerned about how the information will affect his spouse, or that he wants his daughter to make the medical decisions – all issues with practical consequences for the clinician.

2. *Acknowledge the patient's concerns.* Clinicians should explicitly acknowledge whatever is on the patient's mind. This demonstrates that they understand a patient's reasoning as well as their emotions.

3. *Ask for permission to revisit the topic.* Consider saying, "My experience is that people's interest in prognosis can change over time, and so I'd like to be able to check in with you again about this in the future. And you should feel free to tell me if you decide you want more information. Is that okay?"

4. *Explore whether the patient is able to "talk about talking about it."* While a patient may not be willing to hear prognostic information now, they may be willing to talk about when it could happen. Questions such as "Can you imagine when hearing about this information would be helpful?" or "When we have this conversation, what information about the future might be helpful?" are ways to talk about talking about the issue.

5. *Make a private assessment about whether prognosis might change a patient's current decision making.* In some situations, clinicians may feel that a patient's misunderstanding of prognosis is contributing to poor decision making. Here, we recommend negotiating for limited disclosure, or clarifying whether another person, such as the health care proxy, could receive the information to make urgent decisions. With a patient's permission, other family members may be given the information and use it to help them avoid making decisions based on unrealistic expectations. Asking about this might look like, "Is there someone else who I can talk to about these issues?" Or, "I can see you want to take it day by day and your wife seems more like the planner. Might I talk to her about the future?" The key question is, does the patient need the information *now*? If clinicians cannot identify a compelling reason to discuss prognostic information during the current session, then they should follow the patient's wishes.

In exceptional circumstances, when you believe there is a compelling reason for discussing prognostic information and the patient does not identify someone else with whom you may speak, we recommend negotiating for limited disclosure. Start with a statement that explains why you think some information is needed: "I understand that you would rather not talk about prognosis today, and I want to respect that. And it makes it very difficult for me to provide you with the best care. I want to share some reasons that prognosis is important for us to cover today – I think it might influence the decision you are thinking about. What do you think about that?"

In the following table, the patient seems to decline to talk about prognosis, but after exploration is interested in one specific piece of information.

WHAT HAPPENED	WHAT WE CAN LEARN
Dr. T: Are you interested in talking about the prognosis for this kind of cancer? Some people want lots of details, some just want the big picture, and others would rather talk about these issues with their family. What about you?	*Asking the opening question.*
Mrs. P: I know you can't tell me exactly how long I have.	
Dr. T: Well, that's true. The best I can do is give you my best sense based on statistics and averages. And I know that not everyone wants that.	*The doctor is trying to understand why the patient doesn't want to know.*
Mrs. P: Only God knows what will happen to me.	
Dr. T: It sounds like faith is important to you.	*Acknowledging the patient's values.*
Mrs. P: Of course it is! My whole church is praying for me.	*Her coping is linked to her faith.*
Dr. T: It's great to have that kind of support.	*Showing respect for the patient's faith. Privately assesses that she doesn't have to know today.*
Mrs. P: I don't know what I'd do without it.	
Dr. T: You're lucky to have such a strong foundation. Now can I check in about something else? As you think about the future, what concerns you the most?	*Exploring the patient's concerns.*
Mrs. P: I'm hoping that this chemo you've been talking about is going to work.	
Dr. T: I hope so too. Are you open to talking about what we might do if the chemo doesn't work?	*Testing a hypothesis about what information the patient might want to know.*
Mrs. P: Ummm, okay.	

WHAT HAPPENED	WHAT WE CAN LEARN
Dr. T: It sounds like you're not sure if you want to talk about that.	
Mrs. P: Well, actually I do, but what can you say? Isn't this in God's hands?	*She appears to be experiencing a conflict between what she'd like to know and her faith.*
Dr. T: Can I mention something? I think that talking about the chances that the chemo will work doesn't really affect someone's faith. I think you can have a lot of faith and still benefit from the information that we have gotten from clinical trials and research. Some people find knowing about what has happened to other people helps them plan.	*Explaining that knowing prognosis doesn't interfere with faith.*
Mrs. P: That makes sense. So how often does the chemo work?	
Dr. T: Well, the chemo makes the cancer shrink for about four of every ten people that take it. That means that for six out of ten people, the cancer does not shrink. We will check your CT scan after about two months of chemo to see if it is shrinking your cancer. And if the chemo is working, we will continue. If the chemo is not working, and the cancer is growing, then we're in a new situation with different chances. Does that all make sense to you?	*Double-framing the statistical information – talking about the proportion for whom the chemo works, and also the proportion for whom the chemo does not work.*
Mrs. P: You said four out of ten people have their cancer shrink, is that right?	
Dr. T: Yes, you've got it exactly. Is this anything like what you expected?	*Reinforcing the patient's understanding.*
Mrs. P: I'm going to tell my friends at church and have them pray for me and make sure I'm one of those four. I'm worried about this.	

WHAT HAPPENED	WHAT WE CAN LEARN
Dr. T: Of course, all of this is scary.	*Making an empathic guess about the patient's feelings.*
Mrs. P: Yes, it is scary. But I'm glad you told me. Now I know what we are up against and what we need to ask the Lord to do.	
Dr. T: What other questions do you have? Can I check in with you next time about any questions you might have about prognosis?	*Asking permission to revisit the topic.*
Mrs. P: No, I don't have any more questions just now, but I'll be sure to ask you if any come up.	

For Patients Who Are Ambivalent

In our experience, a substantial number of patients do not fit neatly into either wanting or not wanting prognostic information. These patients have mixed feelings about knowing their prognosis: they both want to know and don't want to know. Ambivalent patients can frustrate clinicians because the patient may go back and forth in one visit, wanting the opposite of whatever the clinician proposes. Ambivalence may also be subtle: patients might say verbally that they want to talk about prognosis, but simultaneously give other signals by changing the topic or looking away. The principle for dealing with ambivalence is to discuss it explicitly, allowing patients to talk about both the pros and cons of discussing it.

1. *Name the ambivalence.* Acknowledge that the patient has good reasons both for wanting and for not wanting the information. One might say, "It sounds like you have some reasons that you want to know and reasons that you don't want to know. Do I have that right?" This step demonstrates to patients that we understand their individual complexity and are not going to try to close the discussion prematurely.

2. *Explore the pros and cons of knowing and not knowing.* Rather than trying to push the patient into either category, ask the patient to explain both sides of their dilemma. For example, a clinician could say, "I hear that you have mixed feelings about this, so could you help me understand your feelings – on both sides – in more detail?" As the patient talks, a decision may become clear. Additionally, it may become clear as they talk that they already *know* the essential information about their prognosis (discerned perhaps through their own decline in function); they just may not want to hear more specifics from someone else right then.

3. *Acknowledge the difficulty of the patient's situation.* In our experience, a great deal of ambivalence is rooted in patients' tension between wanting to know information for pragmatic reasons and being fearful of the emotional impact of the information on themselves and loved ones. This tension is not something that a simple communication technique can relieve. We recommend that clinicians first try to demonstrate that they understand the patient's difficult situation and then articulate their willingness to simply be present with the patient. This requires both mindful attention and, verbally, an empathic response. In teaching this, we often observe that clinicians treat the empathy as a clause before an action statement ("I know this is bad, but we can do another test, medication, or chemotherapy"), which undercuts the power of empathy. In these situations, we encourage clinicians to *empathize* with patients' difficult situations and *wait* for patients to initiate the next step in determining how much information they need. At this point, clinician empathy provides the support and safety needed for the patient to face a difficult reality, which is why empathy remains our single most useful communication practice.

4. *Consider outlining the options for a discussion and the consequences of having the conversation.* While empathy enables clinicians to address most ambivalent patients, we occasionally take one further step. In this step, we outline the options for discussion (which are usually different options for disclosure), and the ways in which these options will meet the patient's concerns. Talking about the consequences of the discussion may enable the patient to come to a decision: "I could give you information about the statistical chance that the chemo would shrink the cancer, and that might give you a sense of whether you want to take a trip now or wait until later."

What If the Patient and Family Have Different Information Needs?

What do you do when the patient wants you to be a cheerleader and the family needs the facts? If the wife explicitly asks, "How much time do we have?" while the patient is shaking his head, how can you balance the needs of both? This is especially difficult when being explicit about prognosis with a family member likely includes more information than the patient wants to hear. The key in this situation is to ask each person how much he or she wants to know before you give the information. You could turn to the patient and say, "Your wife would like to hear more about what might happen when you get home, including your prognosis. Is this something that you want to know as well?" If the patient does not want the information, one can say, "Given that you are not really interested in all the information your wife wants, would it be okay if I talk to her separately after our meeting together?" This allows the wife to get the information she needs without burdening the patient. You may also want to tell the wife that it might be hard for her to share the information with the patient, so if the patient becomes curious, he could come back for another visit so you can give the news, to prevent leaving her with the burden of giving serious news.

Discussing Prognosis and Hope

First-person patient accounts of illness are riddled with stories of blunt clinicians who "destroyed hope." When we hear such a story, it is usually the result of "truth dumping" where information is shared without assessing the patient's preference. These experiences lead clinicians to worry about "taking away" hope, yet studies indicate that when families feel that clinicians are responsive to their information needs, resulting conversations can actually make them feel more hopeful. This kind of hope is not so much about a particular outcome that clinicians can bestow; instead, it is about that clinician being present to help the patient face an uncertain future. Your communication task is to show through your responsiveness, empathy, and tact that you are capable of sitting with the hardest situations. That will cultivate the trust your patient needs to talk about difficult prognostic information that no one would want to face alone.

To sustain hope while also helping patients prepare, we find it helpful to frame things in terms of "hope and worry." This allows us to align with patients' hopes while also talking about things we are worried might happen – in other words, hoping for the best, while planning for the worst. For example, to a patient embarking on a chemotherapy regimen with a low chance of response, you might say, "I hope with you that your cancer responds to this treatment and that you are able to get more time. And I'm also worried that you may not be one of the lucky few. Would it be okay if we talk about what we might do if things don't go as we hope?" Or, for a patient with heart failure who is focused on getting stronger despite ongoing decline, you might say, "I see how important getting stronger is to you, and I would also love to see that happen. Given how much things have changed recently, I'm also worried that this may be as strong as you'll ever be, and that things will keep getting harder. Would it be okay if we talk about what we might do if that is the case?"

Navigating Prognostic Uncertainty

While prognosis is never exact, some situations are particularly fraught with uncertainty. Take, for example, the growing use of targeted immunotherapies, some of which can dramatically improve prognosis for some individuals with specific cancers. Or consider late-stage heart failure unresponsive to advanced medical therapies, which is nearly uniformly fatal but for which prognostic uncertainty is such that you might anticipate that a patient will live for weeks or months yet could suddenly succumb to an arrhythmia. How can we tell patients what to expect when we aren't even sure ourselves?

When things are uncertain, clinicians struggle with how to advise their patients, and patients struggle with making plans in the face of an unknown future. So how can we help patients plan in the face of profound uncertainty? Consensus expert opinion now recommends that clinicians talk with their patients about prognosis starting from the time of diagnosis and continuing longitudinally as the illness evolves. Iteratively integrating these conversations into longitudinal care over the course of the illness enables clinicians to incorporate new information – about the illness, treatment options, patient needs and values – and help patients make the best possible decisions as the illness (and the patient's understanding of what it means to live with that illness) evolves.

What might you say when the prognosis is so uncertain that you aren't sure any prognostic information you offer will be meaningful? We find it helpful to name the uncertainty, speaking clearly to both what you do know and what you don't know, as well as identifying the important "what ifs" you really need to talk about to help patients prepare for whatever is to come. You might say something like, "It's impossible to know for sure how your illness will respond to these therapies or how much time you have. I hope that with this treatment we're able to get you more time – several months or maybe even years – and it's possible that may not happen, and that time may be as short as weeks to months. What I can promise is that we'll follow along closely and keep giving you the best information we have as we go, so that we can continue to make decisions together using the best available information." This is also a situation in which "best case/worst case/most likely" language (as mentioned earlier) can be particularly helpful. It provides patients with a range of possibilities that offer some sense of what to expect. Discussing what you do and don't know with patients openly helps them feel supported and trust that you are walking with them to help them with whatever comes.

When the Patient Disagrees with Our Prognosis

What do we do when, after sharing a prognostic estimate, the patient (or family) disagrees and says, "I think I'm going to live longer than that." In thinking about your response, recognize that this may be an emotional reaction and as we've been emphasizing throughout this book, acknowledge the emotions. Also remember that prognostic estimates are predictions about the future and as the patient's clinician wouldn't you be thrilled if you were wrong? Thus, aligning with the patient is never wrong and can help build trust ("I hope you live longer too"). In fact, this may set you up for a future conversation where you can revisit this issue, for example, "While I hope I'm wrong, I wonder if we can think together about what we might do if things don't go the way we wish."

A particularly difficult, and not uncommon, situation is the family that has experienced a prior dire situation in which the poor prognosis didn't come true. How do we respond to the family that says they've heard this before, and we were wrong. It can even feel a bit personal, as if our expertise is being questioned. In response, many of us instinctively want to correct the family's understanding of what was told to them in the past, or explain how this time things really are worse, or even point out that while we were wrong last time, we will be right this time.

Unfortunately, these strategies rarely work. To say, "This time is different," simply invites the same response, "That's what they told us last time." Attempting to correct the family is often perceived as not being heard or, even worse, the medical team not wanting their loved one to get better. Rather than achieving the goal of changing the family's understanding, it leads them to distrust the clinical team and to be even less able to hear what you are trying to say.

We suggest, instead, to start your response with curiosity. The family's statement "That's what they told us last time" may have many different meanings. The family may be confused about how this clinical scenario is different (in which case your impulse to educate them could be correct). Or they may be expressing distrust, given that clinicians were prognostically wrong previously. Alternatively, the family may be seeking to tell us that their loved one is "stronger" than other patients we see and want us to know that statistical predictions are often wrong in his case. Finally, they could merely be saying that, given the previous episodes, they are not willing to change the treatment plan without more data. Since we generally don't know upfront which of these explanations is correct, before trying to "solve" the problem, it helps to get more information, for example, "Can you tell me about exactly what happened last time" or, just "Tell me more."

We also recommend putting yourself in the family's shoes and acknowledging their experience. Acknowledge and even celebrate that we were "wrong" and that the patient has done better than predicted ("I am glad we were wrong before and you got more time with your dad"). Recognize that this family is trying to make the best decisions for their loved one. And, given the uncertainty in medical prognostication, this is very hard to do for anyone. Acknowledging this will help the family feel seen and show that you appreciate that they are doing the best they can. ("I can see you are trying to make the best decision and it's hard because we can never be certain about what the future will hold.") If you think that mistrust is central, it may also help to name this. ("It feels like it is hard to trust us because we were wrong last time about what we thought would happen.") Naming what the family is feeling builds partnership and trust for future conversations. Finally, if you feel a need to give information, check yourself by asking permission – "Would it be helpful if I shared why I think this time might be different?" Asking before telling is respectful and gives the family some control over the conversation.

When Families Don't Believe Our Prognostic Estimate	
Skill	Example
Curiosity	"Tell me exactly what happened last time."
Praise	"I'm so glad he did get better. And, honestly, I'm glad we were wrong the last time."
Naming	"It sounds like it's hard to trust the medical team because last time we said he was not going to get better and we were wrong."
Ask permission	"Would it be okay if I explain why I'm worried that this time might be different?"

These can be some of the hardest conversations. Rather than trying to fix someone else's view, your goal should be to build a relationship. Acknowledging that we would be pleased to be wrong and watch their loved one improve joins us with the family and keeps the door open to future conversations. And you can lay the groundwork for those future conversations by saying, "I hope your dad will do better than I was suggesting. Can we think together about how we'll know over the next day or two if things are moving in the right direction like the last time or if he is going to get sicker?"

These techniques require that we change our role from being an expert to being a supportive guide. Our purpose is less about education and more about acknowledging, praising, and remaining curious while we see what the future brings.

The Bottom Line

Before you talk about prognostic information, spend a minute finding out what the patient wants to know.

Maximizing Your Learning

1. Set aside a few minutes to think about one of the last times you talked about prognosis with a patient. What did you say, and what did the patient say? What did the patient do during the discussion? Did he or she look to a spouse, or begin talking about something else? What did the patient talk about, and what was the intent of that story? And what was the feeling you got from this – both the patient's emotion and yours?

2. Another kind of self-assessment question is to ask your patient: "Have I discussed the future in a way that helped you?" While this may seem similar to the "checking for understanding" step described earlier, this question is meant to focus on the process of the conversation rather than the accuracy of information delivery. Real success in discussing prognosis means engaging the patient in a process of growing understanding about their situation, understanding the patient's evolving information needs, and providing the information in a way that the patient can take it in.

Further Reading

Back, A. L., and R. M. Arnold, Discussing prognosis: "How much do you want to know?" Talking to patients who are prepared for explicit information. *Clin Oncol*, 2006, **24**(25): 4209–13.

Campbell T. C., E. C. Carey, V. A. Jackson, et al., Discussing prognosis: Balancing hope and realism. *Cancer J*, 2010, **16**(5): 461–6. doi: 10.1097/PPO.0b013e3181f30e07. Review. Erratum in: *Cancer J*, 2011 Jan–Feb; **17**(1):68. PubMed PMID: 20890141.

Christakis, N. A., *Death Foretold: Prophecy and Prognosis in Medical Care*. Chicago, University of Chicago Press, 1999.

Jacobsen, J., T. J. deLima, and V. A. Jackson, Misunderstandings about prognosis: An approach for palliative consultants when the patient does not seem to understand what was said. *J Pall Med*, 2013, **16**(1): 91–5.

Jenkins V., L. Fallowfield, and J. Saul. Information needs of patients with cancer: results from a large study in UK cancer centres. *Br J Cancer*, 2001, **84**(1): 48–51.

Lakin J. R. and J. Jacobsen, Less is more: Softening our approach to prognosis. *JAMA Intern Med*, 2019, **179**(1): 5–6.

Rodin, G., C. Lo, A. Rydall, J. Shnall, C. Malfitano, A. Chiu, et al., Managing cancer and living meaningfully (CALM): A randomized controlled trial of a psychological intervention for patients with advanced cancer. *J Clin Oncol*, 2018, **36**(23): 2422–32.

Rosenberg, A., R. M. Arnold, and Y. Schenker, Holding hope for patients with serious illness. *JAMA* 2021, **326**(13): 1259–60.

Temel, J. S., A. T. Shaw, and J. A. Greer, Challenge of prognostic uncertainty in the modern era of cancer therapeutics. *J Clin Oncol*, 2016, **34**(30): 3605–8.

5

Planning for the Future: Discussing What's Important, Well Before a Crisis

How to Start?

Most clinicians would prefer that patients plan for their future illness care in times of calm, before things become urgent or they lose the ability to make their wishes known. Yet only a small percentage of patients actually have these "planning for the future" discussions, and even fewer formalize them into advance care plans. Why is that? Well, most patients would rather focus on the here and now, clinicians can find raising the topic awkward, and even when it's done properly, it's not clear that the results of these early conversations affect the outcomes of care.

Yet many of us sense that when done well, early conversations about goals of care can bring patients and clinicians closer together, provide opportunities to find meaning in illness, and may make future conversations easier when the situation evolves to a point where patients face clear choices. Overcoming barriers to these conversations requires building one's skills and intentionally planning when they will occur.

Many patients want to have these conversations yet expect their clinician to raise the topic. Although less fraught than talking about serious news or prognosis, these conversations can still raise similar emotions as they remind patients that their illness is potentially life-threatening and could lead to difficult decisions down the road. Therefore, our approach to these conversations depends on similar skills.

We would be remiss if we did not also address a recent controversy within the scientific community about the value of advance care planning. An increasing body of literature suggests that early advance care planning (as compared with "in the moment decision-making"), and particularly the advance directive, does not achieve its goal of influencing future medical care. We are sympathetic to this perspective and, therefore, do not recommend early conversations that focus on specific treatment decisions or the completion of advance directive forms. However, we continue to believe that conversations early in serious illness that focus on what matters most to patients deepen relationships, may help guide care decisions over time, and prepare patients, families, and clinicians for future conversations about specifics. It also sets a precedent for multiple smaller conversations over time which may be easier and less stressful than one big one.

Finally, given that choosing a surrogate decision-maker may be the most useful outcome of such a conversation, we strongly encourage early discussions about choosing a health care proxy. Hospitalized patients who have lost capacity and have no identified decision-maker create angst for everyone. Even worse are the cases in which a patient's nontraditional family and biological family disagree and the clinical team is left not knowing with whom the patient would have wanted us to talk. Therefore, early conversations are particularly important when caring for people diagnosed with illnesses that may affect their future decision-making capacity or ability to communicate, such as dementia, primary brain tumors, or neuromuscular diseases, and patients who would want a nontraditional family member to make decisions should they lose capacity.

Yet finding a way to fit such conversations into a busy clinical day can be a real challenge. For clinicians who practice in the outpatient setting with back-to-back appointments, scheduling these patients before lunch or at the end of the day allows space for a bit more time if needed. Some clinicians will schedule a longer appointment in anticipation of needing more time, and new regulations allowing for reimbursement of these discussions make this easier to accommodate. In the hospital setting, we have found it makes sense to have these conversations soon after a recent diagnosis of a serious illness or a discussion of prognosis. Admission to a long-term care facility can also be a good opportunity to gain an understanding of what matters most to a patient. In our experience, it helps to highlight the conversation as part of your agenda for the visit, no matter the setting, so patients know it is something you are planning to address.

The Pitfall: Deferring discussing goals of care and, particularly, surrogacy, until it becomes absolutely necessary.

The Solution: Plan on multiple small conversations over time.

Key Skill: Starting the Conversation with the Patient and Family

A Roadmap for Discussing Early Goals of Care: PAUSE

Pause	
Pause to make time for the conversation.	*"There is something I'd like to put on our agenda today."*
Ask permission to discuss the topic and explain why.	*"Would it be okay if I asked your thoughts on something? Occasionally one of my patients gets sick suddenly and I can't talk to them about it. I worry in these situations that I won't know what matters most to my patient and what care we should provide. Have you ever thought about anything like this?"*
Uncover values first (don't lead with code status).	*"If your disease were to get worse and life might be short, what would be most important to you?"*

Pause	
Suggest selecting a surrogate.	*"Have you ever thought about who you would trust to make your medical decisions if you were too sick to make them yourself?"*
Expect emotion/End.	*"I know conversations about the future can be scary."* (names the emotion)

Step 1: Pause to Make Time for the Conversation

Early discussion about a patient's values and goals is one of those things that can easily get bumped aside by the concerns of the day and acute clinical issues. Setting an agenda helps to intentionally create space for the conversation. When you include it in the plan for the visit, you can make sure it is something that both you and the patient are expecting to discuss in the time that you have.

WHAT HAPPENED	WHAT WE CAN LEARN
Mary G, PA-C: Good to see you today, Ms. Reyes. I know we need to discuss how things are going with your MS treatment. Is there anything you want to make sure we address?	*Setting the agenda.*
Ms. R: I've had some trouble sleeping lately. I guess I'm anxious about my difficulty walking and my neuropathy.	
Mary G, PA-C: Okay. We will definitely talk about those things. ***There's something else I'd also like to put on our agenda today***.	*Reassures patient that her needs will be addressed and alerts her that the clinician also has a topic to cover.*
Ms. R: Okay, what is it?	
Mary G, PA-C: As we work together to manage your MS, I'd like to make sure I understand your priorities, so I know I'm on the same page as you.	*Introduces the topic broadly and in a patient-centered way.*
Ms. R: I appreciate that.	

WHAT HAPPENED	WHAT WE CAN LEARN
Mary G, PA-C: Great we will get to that a bit later. Let's talk about how the medications are going and your concerns first. Is that okay?	*Quickly pivots to the clinical update and prioritizes the patient's concerns.*
Ms. R: Yes, that sounds good.	

Setting an agenda helps you include important nonurgent items, makes sure you aren't missing anything that the patient is concerned about, and helps prevent the "door handle question." Sometimes, as in the example above, the patient's concerns about their illness or new diagnosis may help you segue into the conversation about planning for the future. Setting an agenda can help improve the quality of patient–clinician interactions and can help prioritize issues within the time spent together.

Step 2: Ask Permission to Discuss Goals

When you are ready to transition to talking about goals, asking permission helps signal to the patient that you are changing topics and it allows them a sense of control over the conversation.

WHAT HAPPENED	WHAT WE CAN LEARN
Mary G, PA-C: Would it be okay if I asked your thoughts on something?	*Mary first asks permission to move forward.*
Ms. R: Sure.	
Mary G, PA-C: Occasionally, one of my patients gets sick suddenly and I can't talk to them. I worry in these situations that I won't know what matters most to my patient and what care we should provide. Have you ever thought about anything like this?	*The clinician poses the question in terms that focus on what's important to the patient and maintains a stance of curiosity.*
Ms. R: Honestly, no … I guess I should.	

You'll note that the clinician here uses indirect language. She mentions "one of my patients" rather than the person across from her, which can allow a difficult topic to be less personal and emotionally safer. Using a hypothetical situation allows some psychological distance from the patient's current situation which may make it easier for the patient to engage. This approach can also be used to assess your patient's readiness to engage in conversations about their goals as their disease progresses.

Step 3: Uncover Values

WHAT HAPPENED	WHAT WE CAN LEARN
Mary G, PA-C: If at some point the MS were to get worse and we worried that life might be short, what would be most important to you?	Frames the question around values, not treatments.
Ms. R: Um … I would want to try to get better, but if that didn't work, I'd want to be at home with my family.	
Mary G, PA-C: What else would be important?	*Mary doesn't stop with the first goal and continues to probe.*
Ms. R: I want to make sure that my family is financially secure.	*Reveals new information that could be relevant to future decision-making.*
Mary G, PA-C: Thank you so much for sharing what matters most to you – this will help us guide your care over time.	

In this example, the clinician felt comfortable asking the patient about a hypothetical future state. Raising the question of goals for an extreme situation helps prepare patients to talk about their wishes with clinicians and surrogate decision-makers in the future.

Steps 4 and 5: Suggest Selecting a Surrogate/ Expect Emotion

WHAT HAPPENED	WHAT WE CAN LEARN
Mary G, PA-C: Have you ever thought about who you would trust to make your medical decisions if you were too sick to make them yourself?	
Ms. R: "I think probably my wife … ."	
Mary G, PA-C: The best surrogate is someone who knows you well and can help us figure out what you would want.	*Sensing some hesitancy, the clinician suggests criteria for selecting a surrogate.*
Ms. R: I think she can do it. I trust her.	
Mary G, PA-C: Sounds good. Have you two ever talked about this sort of thing?	*Encourages discussion with the surrogate, as many have never had this discussion.*
Ms. R: No, not yet. Is there something you aren't telling me?	
Mary G, PA-C: I can see this is making you feel concerned.	*Mary recognizes that the patient is worried and names the emotion.*
Ms. R: Yeah. It's just a little scary to consider.	
Mary G, PA-C: I agree it can be scary. That's why I try to talk about these things with my patients when it isn't urgent, so they have time to think and talk to their family and surrogate decision-maker. It's like a fire drill – no one wants or even expects a fire, but it's best to be prepared.	*In response to the worry, the clinician normalizes her practice of talking to patients about these issues.*
Ms. R: That makes sense.	

In this example, the clinician clarifies the role of the surrogate decision-maker as the person who would make decisions in line with the patient's wishes. When the patient expresses concern about discussing a time when her illness may worsen, the clinician responds with empathy, both naming the emotion and reflecting back what was said, showing understanding. Using empathy skillfully in this way helps to build trust and improves the patient–clinician relationship, which is key for future conversations. Remember, you don't have to do it all at once.

Ending the Conversation

In wrapping up the discussion, make sure to acknowledge that these topics can be hard to discuss. We've also found that expressing gratitude for being willing to engage in a tough conversation and ending on a positive note will make it easier to re-engage in the future. Finally, make a plan for next steps.

WHAT HAPPENED	WHAT WE CAN LEARN
Mary G, PA-C: It's not easy to talk about these things.	
Ms. R: No. It's really not.	
Mary G, PA-C: We covered a lot. I really appreciate you being willing to have the discussion. It will help make sure we are taking good care of you the way you want.	*The clinician thanks the patient for engaging in this topic.*
Ms. R: Thank you. I know it's important.	
Mary G, PA-C: Would you like some information to look at as you think about things before our next visit?	*Offers additional resources.*
Ms. R: Sure. I appreciate that, it helps for me to look at information on my own.	
Mary G, PA-C: Great. I'll put a web link in your after-visit summary for your reference, and I'll see you back next month with your wife and we can talk more?	
Ms. R: Sounds good.	

Next steps for the patient may include online resources (listed at the end of the chapter), talking to a surrogate decision-maker or family members, bringing in an old advance directive document, or considering new documentation, as appropriate. Of course, the clinician should document the conversation in the appropriate place in the medical record, have any completed documents scanned, and record next steps as reminder for follow-up by the clinician or a colleague.

What If the Patient Doesn't Want to Talk about Their Goals?

Even if you have all the time in the world and you are motivated to discuss goals early in a serious illness, what if your patient isn't interested? Well, you've collected some very important data and this is still a useful conversation! Now is a perfect opportunity to gently explore the "why" behind that resistance, with the caveat that the primary goal in these situations is to plant the seed and preserve your relationship. Carefully dipping a toe in the water and using a motivational approach may help make future conversations, when they're really needed, easier.

WHAT HAPPENED	WHAT WE CAN LEARN
Clinician: Would it be okay if I asked your thoughts on something?	
Patient: Sure.	
Clinician: Occasionally one of my patients gets sick suddenly and I can't talk to them. I worry in these situations that I won't know the sort of care they want. Have you ever thought about that situation?	
Patient: No, I don't like to think about those things …	*Patient makes her resistant clear.*

WHAT HAPPENED	WHAT WE CAN LEARN
Clinician: It can be a hard thing to think about. Tell me more about that.	*Empathizes with this response and explores.*
Patient: Right now, I'm just trying to stay positive and take it one day at a time. It's too much.	
Clinician: You are dealing with a lot, and focusing on the one day helps it feel more manageable.	*Validates patient's concern.*
Patient: Yeah. I get overwhelmed and then I get really sad. I need to focus on getting better and taking care of my son.	
Clinician: Sounds like being there for your son and focusing on your treatment is what you can handle at the moment.	*Acknowledges the patient's emotional limits.*
Patient: That's it.	
Clinician: Okay. We can come back to thinking about planning for future possibilities at another visit. For today, let's focus on the plan to help you feel better right now. Does that sound okay?	*Keeps the conversation open for a future time while respecting the patient's current emotional state.*
Patient: Yes. That sounds good. Thank you.	

The Bottom Line

Making time to plan and discuss values in times of calm will help patients consider what's most important before a crisis occurs. Helping patients talk to their surrogates about their values allows them to practice these important skills and create a shared understanding before they must make big decisions.

Maximizing Your Learning

Early goals-of-care discussions are important and take a certain amount of conscious effort to get going. Knowing that your primary goal in these conversations is to identify a health care surrogate may make them feel less threatening. Thinking about ways to fit these discussions into your routine and your everyday language for your patients is also a start, as well as recognizing any discomfort you may feel. What is getting in the way of incorporating these discussions early in the disease process for patients in your own practice? Reflect back on a time when you were able to have an early goals-of-care discussion with a seriously ill patient. What helped make that happen? Now consider how you've felt when you've made decisions near the end of life with a patient and surrogate decision-maker who have been prepped with prior conversations. In what ways are they different from those patients who have never discussed the topic? Consider how you might try intentionally focusing your energy on a small number of patients, something achievable, each week. Be curious and see how small wins can generate more success.

Resources

Many resources exist (aside from VitalTalk) for patients and clinicians that may aid them in discussing early goals of care. Here are some examples from communication skills colleagues:

-   Prepare for Your Care: Videos with patient vignettes and online resources for advance care planning that patients can do alone or with their surrogate decision maker. In English and Spanish. Can print advance directives. www.PrepareForYourCare.org
-   Go Wish Cards: Card deck (physical and online) for patients to sort and review with their surrogate decision maker and/or medical provider to stimulate discussion about wishes at end of life. In multiple languages. May be used with people with different cognitive abilities and limited English. www.gowish.org

- ACP Decisions: Video decision aides for patients to watch on a variety of topics including CPR and intubation prior to discussion with their medical provider. In multiple languages. www.acpdecisions.org
- Serious Illness Conversation Guide: Guide for clinicians discussing goals of care with emphasis on prognosis. www.ariadnelabs.org/areas-of-work/serious-illness-care

Further Reading

Back, A. L., R. M. Arnold, W. F. Baile, K. A. Edwards, and J. A. Tulsky, The art of medicine: When praise is worth considering in a difficult conversation. *Lancet*, 2010, **11**(97444): 866–7.

Chochinov, H. M., S. McClement, T. Hack, G. Thompson, B. Dufault, and M. Harlos, Eliciting personhood within clinical practice: Effects of patients, families, and health care providers. *J Pain Symptom Manage*, 2015, **49**(6): 974–80.e2.

Epstein, R.M., T. Hadee, J. Carroll, S. C. Meldrum, J. Lardner, and C. G. Shields, "Could this be something serious?" Reassurance, uncertainty, and empathy in response to patients' expressions of worry. *J Gen Intern Med*, 2007, **22**(12): 1731–9.

Hooper, S., C. P. Sabatino, and R. L. Sudore, Improving medical-legal advance care planning. *J Pain Symptom Manage*, **60**(2): 487–94.

Jackson, V. A., J. Jacobsen, J. A. Greer, W. F. Pirl, J. S. Temel, and A. L. Back, The cultivation of prognostic awareness through the provision of early palliative care in the ambulatory setting: A communication guide. *J Palliat Med*, 2013, **16**(8): 894–900.

Kowalski, C. P., D. B. McQuillan, N. Chawla, C. Lyles, A. Altschuler, C. S. Uratsu 1, et al., "The hand on the doorknob": Visit agenda setting by complex patients and their primary care physicians. *J Am Board Fam Med*, 2018, **31**(1): 29–37.

Parry, R., V. Land, and J. Seymour, How to communicate with patients about future illness progression and end of life: A systematic review. *BMJ Support Palliat Care*, 2014, **4**(4): 331–41.

Pollack, K. I., J. W. Childers, and R. M. Arnold, Applying motivational interviewing techniques to palliative care communication. *J Palliat Med*, 2011, **14**(5): 587–92.

Rodriguez H. P., M. P. Anastario, R. M. Frankel, E. G. Odigie, W. H. Rogers, T. von Glahn, et al., Can teaching agenda-setting skills to physicians improve clinical interaction quality? A controlled intervention. *BMC Medical Education*, 2008, **8**(3).

Sudore, R. L. and T. R. Fried, Redefining the "planning" in advance care planning: Preparing for end-of-life decision making. *Ann Intern Med*, 2010, **153**(4): 256–61.

White, D. B. and R. M. Arnold, The evolution of advance directives. *JAMA*, **306**(13): 1485–6.

Physicians' Views Toward Advance Care Planning and End-of-life Care Conversations, PerryUndem Research/Communication. April 2016 (John A. Hartford, Cambia Health, California Health Care Foundations) www.johnahartford.org/images/uploads/resources/ConversationStopper_ Poll_Memo.pdf.

6
. . . .

Discussing Treatment Decisions
When You're at a Crossroads

In many serious illnesses, after delivering the news or prognosis, and well before late-stage goals-of-care conversations, most clinicians engage in multiple discussions with their patients about a range of treatment decisions. They must summarize a body of biomedical evidence, present choices to the patient, understand the patient's perspective, and together with the patient come to a decision about which option to pursue. This multifaceted process is complex and, in its totality, goes beyond the scope of this book. Still, one thing is clear: discussing treatment options is much more than simply giving information. Many recommendations about discussing treatments seem to assume that clinicians dispense information like a drug, and that more is always better. While information is important, and patients do wish to be informed, offering information alone is too simplistic a guide for clinicians helping patients with difficult decisions.

A huge literature exists on shared decision-making, including how much and what type of information ought to be shared. In fact, considerable disagreement exists among lawyers, bioethicists, and health care professionals. Without entering this debate, we support shared decision-making and believe that no matter where one falls on the spectrum of information requirements, the model itself is strong.

In this chapter, we focus on how to present information needed for shared decision-making and how to engage patients in that process. We will focus on treatment decisions earlier in the course of a serious illness where patients are at a crossroads between reasonable options. In Chapter 8, we will discuss late-stage goals of care for patients nearing the end of life and for whom few effective disease-directed therapies are left.

Our approach in this chapter is based on studies that have examined how patients feel about information, how they absorb information, and how they want to make medical decisions. Although we do not intend to present a comprehensive review of decision-making, we do offer several clear communication tools that, we hope, will make the decision-making process easier for you and your patients.

Information As a Double-Edged Sword

Sound decision-making rests on patients and clinicians evaluating and acting on medical information. Understanding the facts can help patients make decisions that reflect their priorities, motivate adherence, create realistic expectations, reduce anxiety, and promote self-care. Although a minority (10%–20%) of patients don't want to hear all the details, particularly when negative, most patients report that they desire as much information as possible. Nevertheless, research suggests that many patients with life-threatening illnesses do not feel they have been told all that they want to know.

Access to open electronic health records and the Internet have changed how patients obtain information. Many patients come to visits having read a great deal online and perhaps have already read the clinical notes. At the same time, studies show that in the setting of life-limiting illness, information can be scary and even depressing, and many patients find information to be a double-edged sword. Thus, patients still turn to their clinicians as their most important and trusted source. One study found that patients went online primarily to check recommendations and information they received from their health care team, and that patients wanted to develop expertise about their own condition. Clinicians today need to take patient information-seeking into account when discussing treatment options, and realize they are working in partnership with the Internet.

Steering Between Informing Patients and Overwhelming Them

What's the problem with providing lots of information to patients with serious illness? Information about potential treatments and options is loaded with emotional overtones because treatment success and failure may have life-or-death implications. Information overload occurs when heightened emotions leave patients unable to absorb the amount of information that they could otherwise manage in a less stressful moment. Clinicians who do not find the survival statistics surprising, and whose own lives are not at stake, tend to underestimate the effect of stress and assume that patients are taking everything in. In one of our own studies, a patient put it this way: "After he said the 30% [overall survival] he just kept dinging along in his facts, and I was stunned. Literally, my note-taking was completely done. All I wrote was '30%' the rest of the time all over my paper. And I mean, I just couldn't get past that point. I don't know how to describe it."

Involving Patients in Decision-Making

In addition to the question of how much information to share, patients vary widely in how directly involved they wish to be in decision-making. Degner introduced a useful conceptual model that places patients on a spectrum between a paternalistic, or clinician-centered, decision, and a consumerist, or patient-centered, decision. The few existing studies suggest that a substantial number of patients do not participate in the way they would have liked. Interestingly, one recent well-done study demonstrated that clinicians overestimate the degree to which patients want to be involved and that patients who prefer to delegate decisions to their physician are more satisfied with their care. Given this controversy, we think the real issue is to figure out what the patient prefers and match your approach to their needs.

The Roadmap for Involving Patients in Medical Decision-Making

1. *Prepare for the visit.* In Chapter 3, we mentioned the importance of having an appropriate place and time, and the same is true here. In addition, the clinician should come to the conversation aware of the relevant evidence about potential treatments and how it applies to this particular patient. Thinking out loud while sitting in front of the patient is unlikely to improve the patient's comprehension, and can give the impression that the clinician is indifferent or, at worst, incompetent.

2. *Frame the decision to be made.* Start with assessing what the patient knows (remember "Ask-Tell-Ask"?). You may discover critical knowledge gaps to fill before you discuss the decision at hand. When filling these gaps, be aware that treatment decisions often involve a condition that has worsened or an intervention that has not worked, which means you may be back to talking about serious news (see Chapter 3 and the GUIDE roadmap). Once you know that you, the patient, and family are on the same page and any emotions have calmed, you can then clearly describe the decision to be made. For example, consider a case of a patient with vascular disease and one amputated leg who presents with gangrene in the other leg. You might frame the decision as: "The issue we need to decide is whether we should proceed with amputation of your leg." After framing the decision to be made, use the foundational communication skill of asking permission (see Chapter 2) to see if the patient is ready to discuss the decision today. "Is it okay if we talk now about what should be done? Is there anyone else you want to be here when we make this decision?" This signals a transition to the next step of the conversation and gives the patient some control about when and how to begin the decision-making process.

3. *Ask about decision-making preferences explicitly.* Once you have permission to proceed, clarify how the decision should be made. Consider questions like: "When you have to make a significant medical decision, how do you want to go about it? How have you made decisions in the past? Who should be involved? Some people want to hear the pros and cons and decide for themselves, some people want me to make a suggestion and we decide together, and other people want me to make the decision. What sounds right for you?"

4a. For patients who want shared decision-making:

- *Characterize each option*: Don't dwell only on statistics of treatment success. Instead, focus on telling a story about what each path may look like, including the experience of treatment and functional outcomes. Acknowledge uncertainty openly and consider describing best-case, worst-case, and most-likely scenarios. Highlight the differences between the options and the underlying values that might make a person choose one or the other. For example, "Amputating your leg may help you to live longer but, since you already have one amputated leg, amputating the other leg would mean that you wouldn't walk again."

- *Invite patient perspectives*: "Hearing these options and what each may look like, what is most important to you now?" Try to guide the discussion to the underlying values so you're sure the option they choose matches those values. Relevant values are numerous and may include: cure, prolonging life, improving function or quality of life, comfort, achieving life goals, supporting family, or controlling cost. As you help them deliberate, frame the relevant values neutrally. "For some people, living as long as possible is most important whereas for others, maintaining the ability to walk, even if life is shorter, is more important. Which type of person are you?" If they jump to a decision, ask them to tell you how they came to that decision to try to get to the underlying values. Our job is to help patients think critically about the decision, to push them if we are unsure they understood a risk or benefit or if their reasoning seems to be missing a step.

- *Offer to make a recommendation*: Again, ask permission, "Would it be helpful if I made a recommendation?" If a recommendation is desired, frame your recommendation around the patient's values, for example, "Given what you've told me about your desire to live to see your daughter get married and how your large family would help you move around, even if both legs were amputated, I would recommend that we proceed with the amputation." Then check in on what they think about your recommendation. Sometimes further deliberation will be needed, but a recommendation can be a tremendous help in difficult decision-making by relieving the burden on the patient and helping ensure that the treatment path is aligned with patient goals. In some cases, when you have a strong opinion about a particular intervention, laying your cards on the table first (e.g., "In a situation like this we typically think surgery will do more harm than benefit") makes your view clear and may be a more honest approach. Then, invite the patient's response, and see if there are particular values or facts which you had not considered.

4b. *For patients who prefer clinician-led decision-making:* Explain which factors may impact your recommendation and ask permission to explore them. Most patients can weigh in on some relevant factors that will then allow you to offer a recommendation that matches them. If the patient doesn't volunteer additional factors, you can frame a recommendation around the assumed relevant one and ask for assent. For example, "Usually in this situation, we would proceed with amputation to try to help patients live longer, recognizing that it means they wouldn't be able to walk any more. How does that sound?"

4c. *For patients who just want the pros and cons:* Review the options, telling a story about what each path may look like. The "best-case/worst-case/most-likely" language can be particularly useful here. Help identify the values that may inform their deliberation. For example, "As you think about this, the big question is whether it is more important to try to live as long as possible or preserve the ability to walk."

5. *Check for patient understanding.* Whatever type of decision-making is preferred, it can be helpful to check in periodically to ensure you have been understood. A simple way to do this is to ask, "What questions do you have?" Be careful though, because patients do not want to appear stupid and may withhold questions, only to turn to the nurse after the clinician leaves and ask, "What was she saying?" In addition, people from historically marginalized and lower socio-educational backgrounds are less likely to ask clinicians questions. It's better to put the responsibility on yourself and say, "Sometimes I don't do a great job explaining everything. To help me make sure I was clear, could you tell me in your own words what you understand about the treatment options?" Questions that can be answered with "yes" or "no" (such as, "Are you following me?") are somewhat less useful because patients may simply answer "yes" out of politeness.

6. *Establish how the patient wants to proceed with the decision-making process.* "Sometimes people are ready to make a decision, and sometimes they want to think about it for a while, perhaps talk to other people. What is best for you?" The time frame available will depend on the urgency of the decision but, if it is possible, this strategy can help make sure patients don't feel pressured into serious decisions.

In the following excerpt, we've picked up a conversation midway into the visit. Dr. B is seeing a patient with advanced heart failure who is being considered for a Left Ventricular Assist Device (LVAD) as destination therapy. Before the visit, he reviewed the options and expected outcomes. He started the visit by assessing the patient's understanding of the situation and addressing the patient's distress about his rapidly worsening condition. He is now transitioning into discussing the decision.

WHAT HAPPENED	WHAT WE CAN LEARN
Dr. B: So, the issue we need to address is whether to proceed with the LVAD. Is it okay if we talk about that now?	*Framing the decision and asking permission to proceed with the conversation.*
Mr. A: Yes, please. I'm alone on this and need some help.	
Dr. B: Before I start, I want to ask how you want to go about making this decision. Some people want to hear the pros and cons and decide for themselves, some people want to decide together with me, and some people want me to decide what's best for them. What approach sounds right for you?	*Asking about decision-making preferences explicitly.*

WHAT HAPPENED	WHAT WE CAN LEARN
Mr. A: I want your input certainly. I'd like to make the decision together because I need your experience on this.	
Dr B. I think I've got it … [proceeds to give a good explanation of the options]. Hearing these options and what each is likely to look like, what is most important to you now?	*Trying to get Mr. A to consider how each treatment might align with his values.*
Mr. A: I think I'll just go with the LVAD.	
Dr. B: Tell me how you came to that decision.	*Redirecting the conversation to the underlying values.*
Mr. A: I know there are risks and the surgery and recovery might be hard, but living like I am now isn't an option. If there's a chance I could feel better, get back to taking care of my store and maybe be okay for a few years, I guess I need to take that chance.	
Dr. B: Can I comment on what I'm hearing and make a suggestion?	*Asking permission to offer a recommendation.*
Mr A. Please.	
Dr. B: I think you've got a good handle on this. If your goal is to try to feel better, get back to the store and live longer and you're willing to go through the surgery and rehab and all that goes along with it, I agree that the LVAD does the best job of meeting these goals.	*Offers a recommendation centered around the patient's values.*
Mr A. Thanks. I think that makes sense.	
Dr B: Do you think you're ready to move forward with that decision or do you want to talk more with anyone?	*Establishing how to proceed with the decision-making process.*
Mr. A: I think I'm ready. Thanks for your help in thinking this through.	

While we wanted to illustrate how to lay out the decision in the conversation above, the doctor didn't quite get around to using the statistics, and this is a sticking point for many clinicians. We find that statistics illuminate and confuse in nearly equal proportions. Additionally, it is important to know that there are other factors that patients/families often consider (history of "beating the odds," perception from family that the patient has "given up," etc.) that may cause them to be more or less optimistic than the stated statistic. We can, however, endorse two practices. The first is to pick the one or two most important statistics to discuss (see Chapter 4) and to focus on these. The second practice is to double-frame the statistic – that is, talk about the percentage that will be cured, and also the percentage that will relapse. There is some evidence that double-framing helps patients understand better.

Decision-Making Aids That Really Work

The decision-making literature describes many written, computer-assisted, and coach-based self-management aids for patients' decision-making, but they have limited availability and fall outside the focus of our book. We would, however, like to suggest three simple aids that clinicians can use to immediately enhance the quality of their communication. The first is a brief written summary. Described by Tom Smith, the brief written summary is a handwritten single page that the clinician fills out while talking to the patient and that provides a very basic outline of the conversation. We find this to be tremendously helpful in improving patient comprehension. The outline includes the diagnosis, stage (this was designed for cancer), treatment options, outcomes, and side effects. While this is based on the cancer literature, you could modify this outline for most medical decisions.

The second aid uses the best-case–worst-case language we've mentioned earlier in the book, and was developed by a team led by Gretchen

Schwarze and Toby Campbell to help surgeons talk about high-risk surgery. More recently it has been studied to help nephrologists talk about dialysis and neurologists talk about post-stroke interventions. It is similar to the brief written summary but represents the decision in a hand-drawn diagram that outlines two therapeutic options. For each therapeutic option, the clinician draws a vertical line that represents possible outcomes and writes a description of the best case at the top, the worst case at the bottom, and indicates the most likely outcome somewhere at a point on the line that is appropriately closer to the best- or worst-case scenario. The outcomes focus on what the patient would go through and what their life would be like after the intervention. After hearing and seeing these options, the patient is then asked, "What is most important to you now?" to guide the discussion to the underlying values.

The third aid is giving patients an audio recording of the patient–doctor visit. There have been a variety of randomized trials examining the use of audio recordings, and the effects are generally positive. This technique takes almost no additional time, only that of asking the patient permission and turning on the audio recorder. Some recordings even provide simple definitions for medical terms. Although the recording does help patient comprehension and is found to be particularly helpful for family members who were unable to attend the clinic visit, not all patients will appreciate listening to these difficult conversations again. For example, when discussing recurrent cancer or prognosis, the outcomes of giving patients recordings are mixed, because patients find that listening to the recording revisits the trauma and causes more distress.

The Bottom Line

Ask patients how they want to make decisions and try to help ground decisions in the relevant priorities.

Maximizing Your Learning

Choose one skill to work on. As before, commit to practice. For example, start asking patients about their decision-making preferences. Ask yourself the following question: How will I know if I'm doing better? For example, you might leave the visit with a clear view of the patient's preferences about making decisions. You might even ask the patient at the end of the visit how they felt about your asking them about their preferences.

Further Reading

Ariely, D., *Predictably Irrational: The Hidden Forces that Shape Our Decisions*. HarperCollins, New York, 2008.

Chapman, A. R., E. Litton, J. Chamberlain, and K. M. Ho, The effect of prognostic data presentation format on perceived risk among surrogate decision makers of critically ill patients: A randomized comparative trial. *J Crit Care*, 2015, **30**(2): 231–5.

Chewning B., C. Bylund, B. Shah, N. K. Arora, J. A. Gueguen, and G. Makoul, Patient preferences for shared decision-making: A systematic review. *Patient Educ Couns*, 2012, **86**(1): 9–18.

Epstein, R. M., B. S. Alper, and T. E. Quill, Communicating evidence for participatory decision making. *JAMA*, 2004, **291**(19): 2359–66.

Groopman, Jerome, *How Doctors Think*. Mariner Books, Boston, 2008.

Harrington, S. E. and T. J. Smith, The role of chemotherapy at the end of life: "When is enough, enough?" *JAMA*, 2008, **299**(22): 2667–78.

Kaldjian L. C., A. E. Curtis, L. A. Shinkunas, and K. T. Cannon, Goals of care toward the end of life: A structured literature review. *Am J Hosp Palliat Med*, 2008, **25**(6): 501–11.

Lidz, C. W., A. Meisel, M. Osterweis, et al., Barriers to informed consent. *Ann Intern Med*, 1983, **99**(4): 539–43.

Ruhnke, G. W., H. J. Tak, and D. O. Meltzer, Association of preferences for participation in decision-making with care satisfaction among hospitalized patients. *JAMA Netw*, 2020, **3**(10): e2018766.

Schwarze, M. L. and L. J. Taylor, Managing uncertainty: Harnessing the power of scenario planning. *New Engl J Med*, 2017, **377**(3): 206–08.

Smith, T. J., Tell it like it is. *J Clin Oncol*, 2000, **18**(19): 3441–5.

Sox, H., M. A. Blatt, M. C. Higgins, and K. I. Marton, *Medical Decision Making*. American College of Physicians, Philadelphia, 2006.

Taylor, L. J., M. J. Nabozny, N. M. Steffens, et al., A Framework to improve surgeon communication in high-stakes surgical decisions: Best case/worst case. *JAMA Surg*, 2017, **152**(6): 531–8.

White, D. B., N. Ernecoff, P. Buddadhumaruk, et al., Prevalence of and factors related to discordance about prognosis between physicians and surrogate decision-makers of critically ill patients. *JAMA*, 2016, **315**(19): 2086–94.

7

• • • • • • •

Between the Big Events
Dealing with the Things That Surface in the Quiet

Trapped in the Fixing Mentality

Most of this book focuses on pivotal moments in the trajectory of a patient with serious illness. In this chapter we'll shine a light on the negative image – moments between the big events. These conversations are more common than giving serious news or discussing goals of care; they happen all the time between patients and clinicians who are willing to talk about living with a serious illness (and if you are reading this book, you're one of us). This chapter doesn't apply to a patient who has a car wreck, is taken to the ICU, develops multisystem organ failure, and dies there a few days later. The subset of patients we are addressing in this chapter are those who live for some time with the knowledge that they have a disease that will ultimately prove fatal, such as cancer, HIV, advanced liver disease, congestive heart failure, and end-stage renal disease. Patients with these illnesses live, as one put it, "with a sword hanging over your head."

Adjusting to a life of chronic serious illness, also referred to as "coping," is a huge piece of work, and one that leaves many patients feeling profoundly changed. We hear from patients that when not dealing with a critical moment in their illness, they are able to focus on important relationships and priorities that are often very different from the ones they had when they were healthier. The quieter times allow space for smaller, less-threatening conversations about a patient's health, at a moment that may also hold more uncertainty. The spaciousness of the non-urgent times can allow for education, and let clinicians address worries and fears. Patients also tell us that they want to just get back to "normal," whatever that means to them.

The trick for clinicians is to balance helping your patient find a new normal and enjoy a break from crisis mode, while also living with uncertainty. We are not advocating that medical clinicians who deal with serious illness try to be therapists. But what we hear from both therapists and patients is that caring clinicians can play an important role in fostering positive adjustments. Therapists and writers who think about illness in terms of narrative have shown that the stories patients create about their illnesses are incredibly influential, and some stories promote resilience better than others. Clinicians both hear and contribute to patients' stories, and helping them to navigate these narratives can be an incredibly gratifying part of the job. We encourage you to be open to the possibility that a small conversation can have a big influence.

Even so, in the day-to-day, it's easy to find ourselves focusing on the practical issues in front of us rather than the bigger story. The patient with end-stage liver failure who is wondering about his prostate-specific antigen (PSA) level. The patient with interstitial lung disease wanting you to look at a red spot on her ankle (no, it doesn't itch or hurt). The patient who is finishing adjuvant chemotherapy and wants another prescription for lorazepam, which makes you wonder if she is more anxious than you had realized.

These conversations may not be pivotal in the medical sense, but they can be incredibly important, nonetheless. Turning points emerge when you see an opening to learn more about your patient's experience and an opportunity to share some of your clinical wisdom. Or, to just sit with their previously unrecognized anxiety. We don't think this can happen all the time – we want to be realistic about the demands on your time, energy, and attention. But we do want to bring these moments to your attention, because they allow you to bring yourself fully into the therapeutic relationship, and these moments could be the most rewarding ones of your day.

Using Your Clinical Experience to Guide Patients

Along the journey of a serious illness, it's not uncommon to see beaches where the water may seem placid but you know rocks lie just below the surface. At these times, we can check in to see how the patient is doing, normalize the experience, and offer our support. This is different than making a medical recommendation about what treatment would be best. In these situations, you are offering a different framing, or the possibility of a new story about how your patient can live with the consequences of their illness. The steps may sound familiar, as they echo Ask-Tell-Ask and the emotion response skills described in earlier chapters.

1. *Ask the patient about their perspective on a new symptom or concern.* The trajectory of adapting to an illness may be quite different than the trajectory of the disease pathology. (This may require a deep breath on your part, to give you a moment to step back from any irritation you might experience at the seeming irrelevance of the patient's concern.) You may be an expert in the biology, but we are looking here at the patient's perspective and interpretation – even if it is not biologically accurate. So, take a minute to ask how the patient is interpreting the issue. Is it really death anxiety? For example, you might say, "Tell me what's bringing up the PSA test in your mind now? What have you been thinking about?"

2. *Empathize with the emotional content.* We most often begin with an acknowledgment about the impact of an issue ("Given what you are dealing with, it's really normal to be concerned"), although any NURSE statement could work. Give the patient some space to reflect, and consider floating a hypothesis, for example, "What concerns or worries are bubbling up?" Or, ask the patient, "Could you help me understand how you see this?"

3. *Offer your clinical experience as a way of creating new possibilities.* Consider asking the patient if they are interested in hearing about other patients you've treated. For example, you might say, "What have you tried to help get through these moments? … Would you like to hear how other patients have dealt with this issue?" Your invitation and their acceptance signal a different kind of dialogue within the clinical encounter – you are drawing on your repertoire of past stories to give a patient a sense of what is possible. Offering a story in this way is not a promise that it will happen. Make this story distinct from a recommendation (e.g., you should deal with this issue by …). Don't impose your experience on the patient – just offer it.

4. *Follow up by asking the patient what they are taking away.* "What, if anything, can you take away from this conversation that might help before our next visit?" Success is when a patient leaves with some new interpretations, ideas, or possibilities. Or better yet, did the person come away from this conversation feeling bigger or smaller?

A few examples of this roadmap follow. These are not meant to be exhaustive – we intend simply to give you some ideas about what might be possible.

Completing Planned Disease-Modifying Therapy

For Mr. S, a lawyer with colon cancer, coming to the infusion clinic for his last dose of adjuvant chemotherapy was a complex event. On one hand, he was happy to put the side effects of chemo behind him, anxious to get back to full-time work, and looking forward to a vacation. On the other hand, he was also worried about not doing as much to fight off the cancer, and while the infusion clinic took a lot of time, it gave him a sense of security that all these people were working to keep his cancer from returning. For a patient like Mr. S, simply raising the issue gave him a chance to plan.

WHAT HAPPENED	WHAT WE CAN LEARN
Dr. B: Hey, congratulations on your last dose of chemotherapy! You've done a great job dealing with it all.	*Praising the patient (notice how this is different from telling the patient he should be happy) and marking completion as a milestone.*
Mr. S: Thanks doc, it's been tough. But I've gotten through okay – and now it's a little weird to be done.	
Dr. B: Yes, it is tough. Do you have any concerns about finishing up the chemo?	*Acknowledging the patient's experience of "tough."*
Mr. S: Do you mean concerns about the cancer coming back?	
Dr. B: Well, people tell me that concern is always in the back of their minds. I'm wondering about that, or anything else.	*Normalizes patient's reaction.*
Mr. S: It's hard not to think about the cancer returning. I guess I'm just not sure how to feel with the chemo done.	
Dr. B: There are a lot of complicated emotions. Could I mention some other common things that patients of mine have noticed when they finish their chemo?	*Offering clinical experience.*
Mr. S: Yes of course. Like what?	
Dr. B: One thing is that often people have mixed feelings. They're glad to be done, of course, and they're a little nervous about not having chemo because they felt like it was protecting them.	
Mr. S: Actually, that describes me exactly.	
Dr. B: Tell me more …	*Exploring, and offering further conversation.*

This conversation resulted in a bit of clarity for Mr. S, which enabled him to understand his situation, and allowed his doctor to discuss a couple of practical follow-up actions. Mr. S heard the plan for colonoscopy in a few months and follow-up visits every three months; he also got a referral to a physical therapist to learn some abdominal strengthening exercises to compensate for the strength loss incurred by his abdominal surgery. Dr. B used the completion of therapy visit to remind Mr. S of what he could do to participate in best follow-up, and also to address a common post-treatment issue for patients who have had abdominal surgery. In oncology, these issues are now grouped under the term survivorship, which focuses on long-term side effects. (The scope of survivor care goes well beyond the scope of this book, and addresses situations somewhat unique to cancer medicine. The communication issue we are discussing in this chapter is just one survivorship issue.)

Living with Long-Term Side Effects of Therapy

For Margie, a woman with advanced COPD, starting home oxygen put her "in a different place" with her illness. She was grateful that the oxygen allowed her to go out more and remain independent, but she was also a little resentful that she was now "tethered" to her oxygen tank. Her pulmonary clinic nurse practitioner had seen patients struggle with this kind of trade-off before and recognized the initiation of home oxygen as a clinical trigger for a key communication task: asking about living with the side effects of therapy – both physiological and psychological.

WHAT HAPPENED	WHAT WE CAN LEARN
Ann, NP: How have you been doing with the oxygen?	*Asking an open question, but one that is focused on a particular issue.*
Margie: It's helped me. I can go to the store and not worry so much.	

WHAT HAPPENED	WHAT WE CAN LEARN
Ann, NP: What were you worried about?	
Margie: That I'd get half done with my shopping and be so out of breath; then what would I do?	
Ann, NP: I'm glad to hear that the oxygen helps with that. I know independence is important.	*Acknowledging the emotional value of independence.*
Margie: It is, you know. I'm my own person.	
Ann, NP: Some of my other patients tell me that although the oxygen helps them breathe, they also don't like it. Have you had any thoughts like that?	*Offering clinical experience and asking the patient to comment.*
Margie: Well, I don't like the way it looks.	
Ann, NP: How so?	*Exploring (rather than just agreeing) unearths another level of the patient's experience.*
Margie: It makes me look like an invalid.	
Ann, NP: You're feeling that people look at you differently?	*Reframing the self-judgment of "invalid" to something about what other people do.*
Margie: I get some funny looks, all right.	
Ann, NP: I'm sorry to hear that. That doesn't help, does it?	*Acknowledges the emotion.*
Margie: I hate it. And it sometimes makes me wonder if it's worth it, even though it makes going out so much easier.	
Ann, NP: So, you're feeling kind of torn. On the one hand, it makes you feel better physically. On the other, it's been a hard identity adjustment.	*Offers a complex reflection that further frames patient's dilemma.*

WHAT HAPPENED	WHAT WE CAN LEARN
Margie: That's exactly it! What can you do? (Sighs.)	
Ann, NP: Well, I can't change the way it looks. And I also think the oxygen is benefiting you. Unfortunately, what you're experiencing is quite common. I wonder if you'd be willing to talk with our social worker who's had a lot of experience helping patients with this kind of issue?	*Offering resources, like the social worker who may have more time and expertise on this issue.*

This conversation allowed Margie to express her mixed feelings about living with her need for oxygen, both the positive and the negative, and she appreciated that the nurse practitioner let her talk about both and offered support. Ann, NP used her clinical experience and skills of exploring and attending to emotion to get at some of the challenges Margie was experiencing. In doing this Ann helped Margie feel heard and understood, and allowed her to offer a helpful team member's support and expertise.

Dealing with Challenges and Celebrating Progress

For Franklin, a man with renal cell cancer, his surgical treatment left him with chronic flank pain and his chemotherapy resulted in distressing peripheral neuropathy. He was very pleased that his treatments helped him get to remission, but he was also frustrated with how he was treated when he needed to refill his pain medications. His oncologist had seen many of her patients deal with the stigma of long-term pain treatment and recognized this as a trigger for the key communication task of asking about living with the physical, psychological, and social side effects of therapy.

WHAT HAPPENED	WHAT WE CAN LEARN
Dr. K: How have you been doing with the pain medications?	*Asking an open question, but one that is focused on a particular issue.*
Franklin: The pain is tolerable. I can function and help out at home.	
Dr. K: I'm glad to hear that the pain meds help you function better. I know that doing what you can to help your husband is important to you.	*Acknowledging emotional value of being able to contribute at home.*
Franklin: It's very important for my self-esteem and to relieve some stress for Tom.	
Dr. K: Some of my patients tell me that although the pain meds help them function, they also don't like taking them. How does this fit your experience?	*Offering clinical experience, asking the patient to comment.*
Franklin: Well, I don't like needing them.	
Dr. K: Say more …	*Exploring (rather than just agreeing) unearths another level of the patient's experience.*
Franklin: I don't like taking so many pills, and some people assume I have a drug problem, and are really disrespectful. Like when I called my insurance company to ask them about my medication coverage.	
Dr. K: It's really hard to be treated disrespectfully. I've had patients say that they would rather be in pain than deal with the judgment.	*Supporting empathically.*
Franklin: I wish I could go without them and still live my life, but the pain would have me in bed all day. What kind of life is that?	

WHAT HAPPENED	WHAT WE CAN LEARN
Dr. K: I know it isn't easy to deal with the pain even without other people's judgments. In fact, I'm impressed with all you have accomplished and how hard you've been working to be more active despite your symptoms.	*Expression of understanding and acknowledging suffering, followed by respecting effort and celebrating wins.*
Franklin: Thank you. I have come a long way in the past few months.	

For Franklin, this conversation allowed him to express frustration with how others treat him and celebrate the "win" that he has accomplished in feeling good enough to contribute more at home and help his spouse. Dr. K used her clinical experience and skills of exploring and attending to emotion to better understand what Franklin was thinking and feeling. Dr. K acknowledged Franklin's negative experiences, which is important for Franklin to feel heard. Dr. K also paid attention to Franklin's progress. When Franklin shares his regained functional ability and Dr. K celebrates it, it reinforces the win and contributes to Franklin's positive coping. Franklin is like many others dealing with adjusting to life with chronic serious illness and chronic pain, and the skills Dr. K uses honor the whole spectrum of emotion while bolstering Franklin's sense of well-being.

Reinvesting in the Future

For Kate, after experiencing severe viral myocarditis with partial recovery, it brought up something she hadn't expected: she felt stuck. Even though she felt a lot better now, she was left with a significant cardiomyopathy, was on home inotropic medication, and transplant remained an option. She knew the chances that things could get worse were significant and not something she could ignore. She felt like she couldn't just "go back" to her old life. In the example below, Kate's heart failure physician assistant (PA) recognizes the trigger for a query about reinvesting in the future when she says something about living with uncertainty. The clinician's task in dealing with uncertainty now that the acute illness is over is different than when Kate initially presented. The clinician's goal six months ago was to get her through an acute life-threatening illness. Now his goal is to help her live fully in the present – for whatever length of time it turns out to be – while also contemplating the possibility of a heart transplant, a huge but potentially life-altering procedure.

WHAT HAPPENED	WHAT WE CAN LEARN
Kate: I know things are a lot more stable now, and I'm glad to be over the hump. But I'm not sure about what's next.	
Rob, PA-C: Tell me more what you're not sure about.	*Exploring what the patient meant by "not sure what's next."*
Kate: It's hard to explain. After facing all the scary stuff when my heart failed and getting through it, I feel like a different person. I don't think I can just resume my old life. But I feel stuck about what I should do.	
Rob, PA-C: I'm wondering if it's hard to make plans because you're not certain about what could happen with your heart disease.	*Reframing the patient's words to acknowledge the experience of uncertainty.*
Kate: I think that's part of it. It's like I'm waiting for the other shoe to drop. Will things get better on their own? Will I get a transplant and what would that be like?	
Rob, PA-C: Would you say more? …	*Creating a silence that invites exploration by turning toward the patient, looking at her, smiling.*

WHAT HAPPENED	WHAT WE CAN LEARN
Kate: Sometimes my body feels like a time bomb, just waiting to go off.	
Rob, PA-C: That's a powerful image – like you don't quite trust your body?	*Acknowledging the emotion and exploring.*
Kate: Yes, that's it (eyes welling up).	
Rob, PA-C: I could see why you would feel that. I wish I had a pill to fix that one (smiles). Wouldn't that be nice?	*Understanding, then using an "I wish" statement.*
Kate: No kidding.	
Rob, PA-C: I do think there are ways you can learn to live with the uncertainty, though. So that it could feel not so much like a time bomb – more like an occasional unwanted visitor. I have some ideas about this based on what I have learned from other patients – would you like to hear?	*Offering clinical expertise.*

Rob, PA-C has suggested that Kate could work with her feeling of being threatened by uncertainty and eventually live in a different way with it. In doing so, Rob articulates a way forward, yet does not assume he would be the one to do this work with Kate, and in fact, he will refer her to a social worker for this specific issue. This example illustrates how frontline clinicians can uncover a patient's ambivalence about good news, and can introduce additional interprofessional team members who can help meet the patient's evolving needs.

But What about That Sword?

José has finally been doing well with close follow-up from his cardiology team after being in the hospital three months in a row for heart failure exacerbations and recurrent chest pain from small vessel cardiac disease. He is pleased that he is able to spend more time with his grandchildren and just be out of the hospital, even though he continues to have symptoms occasionally. He has talked to his doctors about his medical wishes in the hospital but is hesitant to bring them up for fear he will "jinx" his current state of relative calm. He does find himself worrying about the future and knows that his heart disease will get worse at some point. His palliative care physician, who began seeing him at his last hospitalization and is now seeing him regularly, tests the waters, knowing that these issues are often on patients' minds.

WHAT HAPPENED	WHAT WE CAN LEARN
José: I'm happy that I can get around the house now and that I feel good enough to spend time with my grandkids, especially the little one.	
Dr. P: That's great to hear! What kind of things are you doing with them?	*Celebrate the positive including the details.*
José: The youngest girl likes to play make-believe, so I drink lots of imaginary tea (laughing).	
Dr. P: Sounds like fun!	
José: It's cute. I'm just grateful to be able to spend time with her, she's so smart and funny. Maybe I'll live long enough to see her graduate …	
Dr. P: I'm grateful you are feeling well enough to spend time with her too. What do you think about seeing her graduate?	*Acknowledging positive coping and gratitude; picking up on unrealistic hope and exploring further.*
José: I worry. I try not to think about it, since I'm doing so well, but I know my heart isn't going to last forever.	

WHAT HAPPENED	WHAT WE CAN LEARN
Dr. P: It is hard to think about. Would it be helpful to talk more about your worries with me?	*Naming emotion and inviting more conversation.*
José: Maybe. It's not something I want to dwell on, but I know talking does make me feel less scared.	
Dr. P: Well, I want you to know that we can talk about this at our visits whenever you feel ready. And I wonder if you can then put the worry away when you're at home so you can focus on enjoying your life.	*Offering to be there for future support.*
José: I like that …	

By noticing the ways that José is making progress and coping in a positive way, Dr. P is able to align with him and celebrate the joy in his life. She also noticed his likely unrealistic hope to see his granddaughter graduate, and asked questions to see if he was able to talk to her about his thoughts for the future. Because the physician offered her clinical experience and offered him control over how much he wanted to talk about it, José was able to consider discussing his concerns and ended up deciding to bring his wife to the next visit to talk more.

The Bottom Line

Offering clinical expertise can allow you to guide patients in their healing in uncertain times.

Maximizing Your Learning

1. Which of your clinical experiences could be useful to other patients? It might help to remind yourself what you've learned from your patients that you'd like to share. Think about at what point in the course of a patient's

illness they might be beneficial. Remember that positive stories about what is possible are much more powerful than negative stories about what to avoid.

2. Ask a colleague for some feedback – if you referred a patient to a psychologist or nurse, ask them if the patient seemed prepared for the referral. Then think about the feedback. How was it valuable? Would you ask that person again? Are there other ways you could ask to get more helpful feedback?

Further Reading

Charon, R., *Narrative Medicine: Honoring the Stories of Illness.* Oxford University Press, New York, 2008.

Frank, A., *At the Will of the Body.* Mariner Books, Boston, 2002.

Hewitt, M., S. Greenfield, and E. Stovall, eds., *From Cancer Patient to Cancer Survivor: Lost in Transition.* The National Academies Press, Washington, D.C., 2005.

Jacobson, J., et al., Helping patients with serious illness live well through the promotion of adaptive coping: A report from the Improving Outpatient Palliative Care (IPAL-OP) initiative. *J Palliat Med*, 2014, **17**(4): 463–8.

Kantsiper, M., et al., Transitioning to breast cancer survivorship: Perspectives of patients, cancer specialists, and primary care providers. *J Gen Intern Med*, 2009, **24**(Suppl 2): 459–66.

Kleinman, A., *The Illness Narratives: Suffering, Healing and the Human Condition.* Basic Books, New York, 1989.

Rowland, J. H. and K. M. Bellizzi, Cancer survivors and survivorship research: A reflection on today's successes and tomorrow's challenges. *Hematol Oncol Clin North Am*, 2008, **22**(2): 181–200.

8

Goals of Care in Late-Stage Disease

Uncovering the Big Picture Amidst Fear and Failure

How Do Goals of Care Differ in Late-Stage Disease?

When prolonging life and living an acceptable quality of life no longer seem mutually achievable, we are prompted to modify the goals of care. Discussing such a change begins a process of transition that, however necessary, is also very scary. Cancer care presents the paradigm for these conversations when a patient has exhausted cancer-directed treatment options and faces the need to stop anticancer therapy. For other serious illnesses, the transitions may be more subtle. For a patient with heart failure, the transition might occur when they find themselves bouncing between pulmonary edema and renal failure. For a frail elderly patient with multiple comorbidities, their functional status may have declined so much that just getting to their myriad medical appointments has become too much. In any case, talking about goals of care at this stage of illness forces a reckoning that things are irreparably worse, and is an uncomfortable moment for patients and clinicians alike. In this chapter, we consider situations late in the course of a serious illness where medically effective choices are limited and clinicians seek to help patients and families discuss their goals as their mortality draws near. (Decision-making in other situations has been previously discussed in Chapter 6.)

For many patients, making a conscious, explicit decision to stop disease-modifying therapy often feels like giving up. For clinicians, recommending the discontinuation of disease-modifying therapy also feels like failure. This makes talking about disease progression difficult. As a clinician, you've helped other patients beat the odds (and taken pride in doing so), so what happened here? It's easy to succumb to the self-doubt (even if unconscious): "I must have done something wrong" or, maybe, "I could have done something a little bit better." Either way, it doesn't feel good, and if the patient doesn't want to stop therapy, the clinician is in the uncomfortable position of telling the patient that the treatments to which they had both made a substantial commitment may have been, in retrospect, a waste of time and effort. An oncology fellow told us, "Having a patient say, 'Now *you're* giving up' makes me feel so terrible, on top of my own feelings of defensiveness. It doesn't feel good not to be offering something else." So is it any surprise that clinicians tend to avoid these conversations – and the patients who remind them of their shortcomings?

Because transition conversations are so uncomfortable, clinicians may use strategies to avoid them. Among the most common is to suggest a break from treatment in the hope that the patient will get stronger. Unfortunately, this approach often leads to patients bouncing back and forth between a rehab setting and the hospital without a frank discussion of what is possible.

No matter how important or appropriate it is to shift the goals of care from focusing on the disease to focusing on quality of life, to have that conversation means acknowledging that what we have been doing has not achieved the goal we were hoping for. We worry that the patient's current quality of life is unacceptable, so we have to step back and reevaluate. None of the options are really any good, and facing this invokes disappointment, loss, and sadness. These conversations force patients to confront the failure of medicine ("Why didn't this work for me?"), their own perceived failure ("Maybe I should have chosen a different treatment or different doctor?"), and existential and spiritual crises ("Why is this happening to me? Didn't I pray hard enough?").

These dynamics make talking about goals of care in late-stage disease much more complex than giving serious news. Because it's so hard, the most common approach we see is for clinicians to ignore the actual transition and to jump to interventions that might be invoked at the very end of life, such as cardiopulmonary resuscitation (CPR) and mechanical ventilation. At the end of the chapter, we'll talk about dealing with code status. But first, we want to describe an approach to talking about goals more broadly, separate from resuscitation, because our recommended approach is to understand values and goals before offering a plan.

> **The Pitfall:** Keep cheerleading until you decide it's time for the patient to be "realistic."
>
> **The Solution:** Work on the big picture and focus on goals that are achievable within the constraints of the illness.

Another thing we see clinicians do rather than deal with the transition is maintain that "Everything is okay" until they say that "Nothing more can be done." Understandably, this abrupt pivot makes it much more difficult for patients and families to wrap their heads around what has changed. Research indicates that patients want to negotiate when to talk about dying and to have some control over the process. They also harbor painful memories of being told that "There is nothing more we can do," a phrase that should always be avoided.

The strategy of redirecting hope from living longer to looking toward a "good death" (as if such a thing were desired, or even regularly achievable) is widely known but often used ineffectively. We find that without a substantial understanding of the patient, simply recommending a shift in goals often fails. To your patient, hearing that he should have new goals sounds simplistic and looks expedient. Our experience is that shifting goals is most successful when it evolves from patients' values, and this takes some exploration. Just as reassurance works best only after you have learned the patient's real fears, redirecting goals is most successful when you have a sense of what is truly important now and what hopes the patient is giving up. In addition, you need to emphasize that the patient will continue to have access to your expertise and that you are not simply pushing them off to hospice. You can't change the reality the patient faces. What you can do is to create a conversation that will provide medical expertise, support, and understanding so that in that moment, the patient can think clearly about the changes and decisions they are facing.

Key Skill: Constructing the "Big Picture" View with the Patient and Family

A Roadmap for Discussing Goals of Care in Late-Stage Disease: REMAP

Before you start down the road of talking about new goals of care, remember the skills you have learned from the previous chapters ...

1. *Prepare yourself.* These conversations are tough, and the more you have been able to think through the case, and come to terms with your own feelings, the better you will be able to hear subtle cues and respond to what is happening in the moment.
2. *Make sure you know where to start.* Often this discussion represents serious news, so recall those skills (Ask-Tell-Ask) and make sure you've asked your patient what they've been told about their illness. That way, you know where to start and what medical information you may need to confirm or convey.
3. *Ask permission (and signal a change in the conversation).* Asking patients if you can move forward with the conversation allows them a sense of

control, and also signals to them that something new is going to be discussed: "Would it be okay if we discussed what is going on now with your medical condition?" Once you understand what they know, and they have given permission, you are ready to move the conversation forward.

4. *Attend to the emotional track.* Because this conversation is about the current treatments not working the way we had hoped and planning for a future that is likely to include further loss and death, emotions may be high. Make sure you are tracking both the cognitive and emotional information that is being conveyed and if the emotions run high, slow down and acknowledge them.

Remap	
Reframe why the status quo is no longer working.	*"We're in a different place … "*
Expect emotion, respond with empathy.	*"You have worked so hard to do everything right."*
Map out big-picture values, what's important.	*"Given this situation, what is most important for you now?"*
Align yourself and the team with the patient's values.	*"It sounds like the most important things to you are your family, being comfortable, and knowing what to expect. Is that right?"*
Plan medical treatments to match the patient's values.	*"Would it be okay if I offered a recommendation on what to do now based on what you've told me?"*

Now let's look at each of these steps in more detail.

Reframing why the status quo isn't working is its own piece of serious news. Be ready with a headline (see Chapter 3).

- *"The scans show that your cancer is growing despite the chemo, and the oncologist thinks that further treatment would cause more harm than good."*
- *"Even with maximal medical treatment, your mom's body is getting weaker, and I worry that she's dying."*

Reframing may also be confirming that they have the information correct.

- *"You have a good grasp of what's happening. We're in a different place now with your heart disease."*

Expect emotion. People will have an emotional reaction to the reframing of their situation. As with other serious news, responding with empathy will often require you to give space with compassionate silence followed by verbal expressions of empathy using NURSE statements. (See Chapter 3 for more on empathic responses.) Sometimes people are relieved that someone is finally talking to them about their situation. At other times, patients and family may harbor mistrust about the medical team and what you are telling them. The good news is that by expressing empathy, you may build trust.

One should ask permission to move forward and discuss the plan, with a question such as "Would it be okay to talk about what we should do next?" If the patient responds to this question with emotion or if the emotion does not dissipate after several minutes of attending to it, the rest of the conversation needs to wait until another day.

To begin to move toward a plan, you should intentionally step back to explore the patient's values before discussing therapeutic choices, for example, by saying "In order to figure out the best plan for you, let's talk for a couple of minutes about what is most important to you at this point."

Mapping out the patient's values allows clinicians to empower patients or their surrogates and creates a shared understanding of the patient's goals before moving to treatment options. The conversation that follows does not immediately focus on treatments. Instead, the clinician explores what matters most to the patient and their concerns about the future. This information helps the clinical team propose a plan that is most likely to achieve the patient's goals given the new medical situation. Too often, we start talking about code status or hospice before we really understand where a patient and their family are coming from.

And you may need to hear from more than one person – such as family members – to understand what the core issues really are. People often make decisions with input from others, so asking the other family members in the room what they value may help make a more complete plan as they likely have different things that they are concerned about.

The Pitfall : Mapping out the patient's values and ignoring the family.

The Solution: Make sure to ask what the family members think is important, as well.

Mapping questions:

"Given this situation, what is most important for you now?"

"As you think about the future what do you hope for?"

"What else?" (repeat)

"What brings you joy or meaning?"

"As you think about the future, what worries you? What are your biggest concerns? What do you want to avoid?"

"What is the hardest part for you? For your family?"

These questions help identify what is valuable and meaningful to this patient and their family, as well as sources of concern. If focusing the conversation on the patient's current illness feels too threatening, a less scary opening could be to ask about the existence of a living will or if the patient had ever thought about what would be important if they got sicker. That said, we tend to shy away from this approach as most patients struggle to answer abstract questions about values. Asking directly about the patient's hopes and worries usually elicits more information.

As tempting as it may feel, we urge you to refrain from commenting on the feasibility of goals or hopes – use this part of the conversation to appreciate and align yourself with the person. For example, if your patient says simply, "I want to live," you can respond "I'm hoping for the same thing for you. Tell me what about your life is most valuable right now and most makes you want to live?" If the answer is "curing the disease," acknowledge that hope, then ask, "Is there anything else?"

The Pitfall: Incomplete mapping, only asking one or two questions about a patient's values.

The Solution: Continue asking mapping questions until the patient runs out of things that are important.

Stopping after hearing the first or second value expressed by the patient may lead you down the wrong path, as you may think you are suggesting a plan that matches what's most important to the patient when, in fact, that plan may actually contradict a value or goal they haven't yet told you (e.g.: (1) No pain, (2) Out of hospital (3) Want a second opinion …). The key skill is to simply keep asking "anything else" after the patient expresses each item of importance, until they signal they are done ("I think that's it"). In most cases, you want to hear at least three things of importance to the patient before moving onto the next step (Aligning).

Key Skill: Eliciting Meaning and Values

Many skills can help clinicians uncover their patients' values and concerns. As we first learn them, we may write down and tuck away the exact words or phrases we see our mentors use, but often we aren't sure how or when to use them. Like a skilled craftsman, over time and with careful observation we learn which tools suit which situations best.

Useful tools	When/how to use it	To what purpose
"If your disease were to get worse and life might be short, what would be most important to you?"	When you want to start to explore your patient's values.	To help your patient consider a hypothetical future state, clarify their values, and practice having goals-of-care conversations.

Useful tools	When/how to use it	To what purpose
"What else is important?"	When you want to map additional patient values.	To make sure you have all your patient's goals on the table – even ones that conflict or are unrealistic. This allows building a better understanding.
"What worries you?	When you want to understand not only what is important, but also things to avoid.	Flipping the questions to worries opens the door to an additional group of concerns that may be important to your patient.
"What do I need to know about you as a person to give you the best care possible?"	When you want to acknowledge your patient's personhood rather than their illness.	To learn about what is meaningful to your patient, build trust, and help the patient know that the clinician sees them as more than their medical diagnosis. This also helps to address cultural differences.
"If you could accomplish what you are hoping for, what would that look like?	When a patient is talking about hopes that are unrealistic.	By not trying to talk people out of their hopes, it allows you to align with the patient on the realistic ones.

Align. Once you feel mapping is complete (e.g., at least three goals elicited) and the patient has shared all of their hopes and worries, you can demonstrate alignment with your patient by reflecting back all of these values and goals. For example, "It sounds like the most important things to you are being comfortable, being out of the hospital, and making sure that there aren't other treatment options. Is that right?" This does a few things. It shows that you listened and heard them. It also gives your patient a chance to correct you if you got something wrong or misunderstood. And, finally, it allows the patient to add something they forgot.

Offer a recommendation. Notice that we ask for permission before suggesting a plan. "Now that I understand more about your situation, would it be helpful for me to make a recommendation?" Asking permission allows the patient a sense of control and helps signal that the conversation is moving forward again. The more you can engage the patient, the better they will hear the recommendation.

As a clinician, your job is to match appropriate treatment options to what's most important for the patient, so that you can best help them achieve these goals. This requires listening intently and then giving a recommendation based on what you've heard. Some clinicians worry that to do so takes away patient autonomy. ***We believe that exactly the opposite is true.*** Patients are looking for a recommendation from their clinician, and they have the power to accept or reject this advice. Remember – your recommendation is not based upon what you would want for yourself. Instead, it reflects what patients tell you is important to them. All of this book's authors have made recommendations for treatment that we would never wish for ourselves, because it was clear that, for that particular patient, the intervention (however aggressive or incongruous to us personally) was consistent with their goals.

Some pointers when offering a recommendation:

- First talk about the things you will do (e.g., pain control, home health services) before talking about what you recommend stopping or not doing (e.g., chemotherapy, CPR).
- Be transparent about conflicting goals (e.g., being full code, dying peacefully at home), if they exist, and enlist the patient's support in resolving.
- Link your recommendations to the patient's stated values ("Show your work").
- Check in for the patient reaction to your recommendation.

The following example illustrates some of these points. We are joining this conversation in midstream – after Dr. B has spent time going over the scans, sharing the news that treatment is not working, and dealing with the sadness. At this point, Dr. B and Ms. T have decided to move on and talk about what is next.

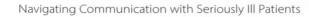

WHAT HAPPENED	WHAT WE CAN LEARN
Dr. B: I know it's hard to get your head around this new information. I want to make sure we take good care of you, and that what we do matches your priorities. So, given what you now understand about where things are at, what's most important to you? [three seconds silence]	*Acknowledging difficulty of the topic. Suggesting a way into discussing the topic. Giving silence as space to allow the patient to decide if she can talk about this.*
Ms. T: What's important, you're not going to be able to give me, though. What's important to me is watching my son grow up.	
Dr. B: Tell me more …	*Explicitly asking to hear more about this – the patient is outlining the big picture issues.*
Ms. T: Watching my kid play soccer – that's his new thing. Just doing normal mom stuff. Plus, what do I go home and tell my husband?	
Dr. B: [three seconds silence]	*Giving more silence as space to allow her to think.*
Ms. T: I'm worried about how my family is going to deal with this.	
Dr. B: Sounds like trying to do normal stuff with your son for as long as possible, and taking care of your family through this are both really important.	*Offering a reflection about the situation lets patient know he's heard what she's said.*
Ms. T: Yes. And I don't know where to start.	
Dr. B: It can sometimes feel overwhelming. We'll talk about some things that may help. What else is important?	*Acknowledges the emotion, briefly commits to helping with this concern, then continues to uncover values.*
Ms. T: I don't want to suffer with a lot of pain, but I want to be alert if I can be.	
Dr. B: Okay. What else?	*Gathering more values.*

WHAT HAPPENED	WHAT WE CAN LEARN
Ms. T: I'd like to live as long as I can, but I'd like to try to stay out of the hospital.	
Dr. B: Both of those make sense. What else is important? Or are there things that worry you?	*Continuing to map values in different ways.*
Ms. T: No, those are the main things.	
Dr. B: Okay. Let me see if I heard you correctly. Living for as long as you can, as normally as you can, which includes good symptom control, is important. I also heard that spending your time with your family outside the hospital and making sure they have support is really important. Did I miss anything?	*Aligning with her values.*
Ms. T: No. You got it right.	
Dr. B: Would it be okay if I made some recommendations about next steps?	*Asking permission to make a recommendation.*
Ms. T: Okay. That would be helpful.	
Dr. B: Given what you've said is important, I can help you talk to your husband if you'd like. I'm happy to answer his questions either in person or by phone. We'll adjust your medications when needed so that we control your pain without making you too sleepy so you can spend good time with your son. We'll treat you for the things that are reversible, like infections if you get them, to try to help you live for as long as possible. There are also some services at home we can talk more about that may help you stay out of the hospital. How do those things sound?	*Give your recommendations, starting with the things you will do, linking them to the patient's goals. Check in to see if the patient agrees.*
Ms. T: That all sounds good. It's a place to start.	

WHAT HAPPENED	WHAT WE CAN LEARN
Dr. B: I also think there are some things we shouldn't do … Whenever your body gets so sick that you are close to death, I think we should not do CPR or put you on a ventilator in the ICU. It wouldn't fix your cancer, and it could cause you distress and would keep you from being home. What do you think?	*Give your recommendations about things to avoid, linking them to the patient's goals. This may be the time to make a recommendation about code status. Check in to see if the patient agrees.*
Ms. T: I think that's right. I don't want to be kept alive on machines or die in the hospital if I can avoid it.	
Dr. B: Okay. My team can help you with documenting that, so that we make sure we follow your wishes.	*You should offer information about legal documentation of the patient's wishes as per your state's requirements.*
Ms. T: Thank you.	

By starting with the things you **will** do, it allows patients to hear that you are going to actively continue to care for them based on their wishes. If you start with all the things you aren't going to do, the patient may feel abandoned or take it as another piece of serious news, and they may not be able to hear or process what you want to do to help because of their emotions.

Hospice may be an important part of many of these new treatment plans. Detailing the services that hospice provides first and then naming the collection of services as hospice may help with the introduction. This is because many patients and families hear the word "hospice" as another piece of serious news and will experience a strong emotional response. By talking first about how the services will meet the patient's needs and goals better than other options, they may be able to hear what the benefits of hospice are before their emotions make it hard to process new information. Either way, you will need to respond to the emotions that come up, but the work is different as the information you have already provided may help create an emotional landing that feels safer. If it applies, make sure to point out how you will still be part of the team.

CODE STATUS RECOMMENDATIONS ARE DERIVED FROM DISCUSSIONS OF VALUES AND GOALS, NOT THE GOAL OF THE DISCUSSION ITSELF

By including code status recommendations as part of the plan based on the patient's values, we allow patients to see why the recommendation is being made, rather than coming out of left field and talking about a disembodied heart and lungs as objects to be restarted, or graphic descriptions of cracked ribs and punctured lungs that may feel coercive. By first discussing their medical reality and their values, we allow patients to see resuscitation as part of the bigger collective of medical decisions to be made to reach their goals. Finally, talking about how someone wants to be cared for when their disease progresses and they approach death feels very different than what is often perceived as a question of "Do you want to live?"

It's also helpful for clinicians to check in with themselves before discussing code status. Emotional trauma and moral distress from difficult resuscitations of patients in your past may affect how you discuss code status with patients now. Taking a moment to see each situation anew will help you be present and listen, so you can make a code status recommendation based on **this** patient's values and medical situation.

Patient Responses to Goals-of-Care Conversations

In our experience, patients respond to these conversations in several ways: they accept the clinician's assessment that a transition is occurring; they want to negotiate; or they decline the clinician's assessment. Alternatively, they accept the clinician's assessment of the situation, but reject the recommended plan.

Patients who accept that a transition is occurring are ready for specific end-of-life planning. You can sense this when patients articulate that they understand the situation, state that they are ready to hear more, and ask questions about what will happen next and what they should be ready to do. These patients are ready for intensive planning and explicit discussions.

Patients who want to negotiate perceive that they are close to a transition but want to see more evidence. These patients, in our experience, tend to raise questions about the clinician's assessment and want to discuss the situation with others – including clinicians, family members, friends, or spiritual counselors. For these patients, we recommend you engage the patient and family in a discussion of clinical milestones. The most useful milestones are markers of disease progression that the patient and family will recognize as independent of clinician judgment (a CT scan measuring the size of metastatic lesions). The next step is for the clinician to construct a time-limited trial of medical therapy using the milestones to judge success (e.g., another month of chemotherapy followed by a CT scan). We find that this process can enable patients and families to step away from concerns about clinician judgment and commitment ("Are they just giving up on me?") and toward a realistic assessment of their situation.

Patients who reject the clinician's assessment that a transition is occurring, in our experience, appear undecided, quizzical, or unengaged. Some withdraw from the conversation, which clinicians may miss as a sign of rejection, and move straight into a discussion about end-of-life planning. Many patients who decline will not articulate this directly to the clinician – they do not wish to confront, contradict, or disagree. They tend not to participate in end-of-life planning that follows – for example, they will listen to a discussion about hospice, but when the nurse arrives will decline to sign up. These scenarios breed distrust and waste everyone's time, so it is worth being very clear about where the patient is at before moving on to the next steps.

In our experience, the most common reason that patients decline the clinician's assessment is that the prospect of current approaches not working is just too sad, too frightening, or too threatening. This is often labeled as "denial" and, indeed, it may be. But, if they are in denial, it is because accepting the truth is too difficult psychologically. These patients are the ones whose responses tempt clinicians to "confront them with the truth," "hang crepe," and "hit them over the head with it" – mostly because the clinicians are frustrated. In these situations, we find that the most useful communication tool is to pay attention to the emotion data and ask about it. Over a series of conversations, patients may be able to explore, tolerate, and understand emotions that they could not otherwise face. What clinicians do to be successful at this point is probably beyond any particular phrase or approach. The clinicians whom we admire rely on attention to subtle patient cues, highly calibrated self-awareness, and complete authenticity. We often hear clinicians speaking of the need to give patients "more time." While we agree that patients may need more time, we think it is helpful to remember that the time they need is time exploring their feelings and concerns – either with us or with another person with the necessary skills.

Finally, patients may agree with our assessment, but not agree with our proposed plan. We discover this when we ask, "What do you think?" about the plan and we get a response such as, "Oh no, you have to try to restart my heart!" The best way to respond to these responses is curiosity. ("Tell me more.") That will help you understand if the issue is an emotional one ("I just can't imagine not being there for my daughter"); a misunderstanding about the medical treatment ("Why can't you restart my heart without me being on a breathing machine?"); or if there are values which you have not elicited ("I want to do everything to stay alive until my great granddaughter is born next month"). Only by being curious and gathering more data can you figure out the best response.

Common Challenges

Patient and family response	Skills to try	Example
"I want you to do everything!"	Respond to the emotion and explore what "everything" means.	*"This must be really difficult to hear. Tell me more about what you mean by 'everything.'"*

Patient and family response	Skills to try	Example
"There must be something more you can do!"	Use "I wish" to align with the patient's hope and avoid discussion of ineffective options.	"I wish there was something more we could do that would help treat the cancer."
"What about a clinical trial? Or a second opinion?"	Don't assume these are real questions that require a cognitive answer. First address the emotion, then pause to see the patient's response.	"This information must be hard to hear after all you've been through."
"We're praying for a miracle."	First, align with the patient's hope. Saying you want the same thing they want does NOT mean that you believe it's attainable. Then, use "and" rather than "but" to introduce options if the miracle doesn't occur.	"I share your hope for a miracle … and I want to make sure we plan for the other possibilities, so we take good care of her no matter what happens. Would that be okay?"
"Our family just doesn't know what to say; we feel conflicted."	If the patient is not available to speak for themselves, bring the patient "into the room" to help the family with decision-making.	"If your dad could see himself right now and understand what is happening and what the future likely holds, what do you think he would say?"
"My daughter is a fighter."	Acknowledge the emotion and explore values using the fight language. Or, redirect the "fight" if possible.	"Clearly she is a fighter. Can you tell me more about what she's fighting for? What's most important to her?"

Patient and family response	Skills to try	Example
"I think it's too soon to make a decision and my brother deserves a chance."	Offer a time-limited trial of continued treatment (or new therapy if appropriate) and engage the family in monitoring for effects of the trial.	"Okay. Let's see how he does over the next two days as we continue maximum medical support for his stroke. And perhaps we can talk about what we'd expect to see if he's improving, getting worse, or staying the same."

Each of these examples may surface feelings in the clinician as well, so take a minute to pause and check in with your own emotions and automatic assumptions based on past challenging experiences (e.g., *Oh no! Not miracle talk. These families are always difficult to deal with*). Take a breath and try to allow each person and family to have their own encounter where you can be curious and hone your skills, rather than fall into dysfunctional patterns and create a self-fulfilling prophecy.

The Bottom Line

A transition to end-of-life care is a turning point in a life – a big, scary, hairy one. Patients and families may not remember the exact words you used, but they will remember your compassion, respect, and empathy.

Maximizing Your Learning

Conversations about goals in late-stage disease often bring up feelings of helplessness, being out of control, and grief for things lost. These powerful emotions are uncomfortable to be with for a clinician, but your willingness to allow these to be present gives a very powerful signal that you're able to talk with the patient about what's really important and can be present with the emotion – which is therapeutic in itself. Think back to an emotionally powerful conversation you had with a patient. What were the feelings that you can remember? (We often find many feelings rising and falling through the course of an important conversation.) Which feelings could you hold easily? Which feelings were tough – that perhaps you really wanted to get away from, or fix, or stop? Identifying these difficult-to-be-with feelings can help you locate your learning edge in goals-of-care discussions. Don't forget to notice, however, the feelings you were able to hold – what happened for the patient because you were able to be present for these emotions?

Further Reading

Back, A. L. and R. M. Arnold, "Isn't there anything more you can do?": When empathic statements work, and when they don't. *J Palliat Med*, 2013, **16**(11): 1429–32.

Back, A. L., S. B. Trinidad, E. K. Hopley, and K. A. Edwards, Reframing the goals of care conversation: "We're in a different place." *J Palliat Med*, 2014, **17**(9): 1019–24.

Back, A. L, S. M. Bauer-Wu, C. H. Rushton, and J. Halifax, Compassionate silence in the patient-clinician encounter: A contemplative approach. *J Palliat Med*, 2009, **12**(12): 1113–17.

Childers, J. W., A. L. Back, J. A. Tulsky, and R. M. Arnold, REMAP: A framework for goals of care conversations. *J Oncol Pract*, 2017, **13**(10): 844–50.

Deep, K. S., C. H. Griffith, and J. F. Wilson, Communication and decision making about life-sustaining treatment: Examining experiences of resident physicians and seriously ill hospitalized patients. *J Gen Intern Med*, 23(11): 1177–82.

Flint, L. A., D. J. David, and A. K. Smith, Rehabbed to death. *New Engl J Med*, 2019, **380**: 408–09.

Leiter, R. and J. A. Tulsky, Willing to wait for it: Time-limited trials in the ICU. *JAMA Intern Med*, 2021, **181**(6): 795–6.

Meier, D. E., A. L. Back, and R. S. Morrison, The inner life of physicians and care of the seriously ill. *JAMA*, 2001, **286**(23): 3007–14.

October, T. W., Z. B. Dizon, R. M. Arnold, and A. R. Rosenberg, Characteristics of physician empathetic statements during pediatric intensive care conferences with family members: A qualitative study. *JAMA Netw*, 2018; **1**(3): e180351.

Pollak, K. I., R. M. Arnold, A. Jeffries, et al., Oncologist communication about emotion during visits with patients with advanced cancer. *J Clin Oncol*, 2007, **25**(36): 5748–52.

Quill, T. E., R. M. Arnold, and F. Platt, "I wish things were different": Expressing wishes in response to loss, futility, and unrealistic hopes. *Ann Intern Med*, 2001, **135**(7): 551–5.

Quill, T. E. and R. Holloway, Time-limited trials near end of life. *JAMA*, 2011, **306**(13): 1483–4.

Rabinowitz, T. and R. Peirson, "Nothing is wrong, doctor": Understanding and managing denial in patients with cancer. *Cancer Invest*, 24(1): 68–76.

Reinke, L. F., et al., Transitions regarding palliative and end-of-life care in severe chronic obstructive pulmonary disease or advanced cancer: Themes identified by patients, families, and clinicians. *J Palliat Med*, 2008, **11**(4): 601–09.

Schofield, P., et al., "Would you like to talk about your future treatment options?" Discussing the transition from curative cancer treatment to palliative care. *Palliat Med*, 2006, **20**(4): 397–406.

Tulsky, J. A., R. M. Arnold, S. C. Alexander, et al., Enhancing communication between oncologists and patients with a computer-based training program: A randomized trial. *Ann Intern Med*, 2010, **155**(9): 593–601.

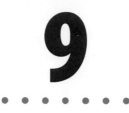

9

Conducting a Family Conference

Reading the Room Under the Light of Group Dynamics

When Does a Family Conference Make a Difference?

How you interact with a patient's family can make or break the relationship you have with the patient. Plus, the family can help you: they can serve as an extra set of ears, reinforce your message, and clue you in on what's important. In the hospital, seriously ill patients often lose decision-making capacity and families serve as their surrogate decision-makers, a role associated with anxiety and posttraumatic stress disorder. Effective family meetings help the family cope better, be more effective caregivers, and feel better supported in their efforts.

An effective family conference can get everyone on the same page, ensure that the patient and family understand the medical situation, and help the family and care team come together to make treatment decisions that align with the patient's values. Most often, family conferences happen in the hospital, but this is also a tool you can use in an outpatient clinic. Family conferences take time, commitment, and a lot of people and, unfortunately, no research tells us when, exactly, this effort pays off.

So, when do we think family conferences are worthwhile? Perhaps the most common trigger is when we need to discuss serious information or medical decisions (e.g., transitioning the goals of treatment from life-prolonging to comfort-focused) and the patient either wants the family involved or is too ill to participate. Another trigger occurs when the patient is unable to participate in decision-making and family members disagree about what needs to be done.

We're not saying that you should talk with family members only in these situations. In fact, for incapacitated patients in the ICU, critical care guidelines recommend that one have a family meeting within the first 48 hours of admission and routinely thereafter to ensure the family is kept up to date and their coping assessed. The roadmap we describe here is useful for all encounters in which family members are involved. However, in this chapter, we focus on the "big" family meetings where you are trying to get multiple family members together, provide information, and determine the overall goals of therapy.

One more note: we use the term "family" to refer to all people the patient loves and wants involved in their medical care. Thus, a patient's "family," for our purposes, may include an unmarried partner, a close friend, or a second cousin – in addition to a spouse, child, or parent.

While family conferences are well established as a communication tool, we have seen them conducted skillfully and poorly with nearly equal frequency. For every clinician who views the family conference as a panacea, another wearily disagrees, asserting that it will yield little progress. So, what can we do to maximize the value of the family conference?

The principles for talking to family members remain the same whether there is one family member or many. However, meeting with a group of people raises some unique issues we have not yet discussed elsewhere. Multiple family members means multiple perspectives, agendas, emotions, and values. Additionally, when patients are unable to speak for themselves, clinicians and families may need to navigate surrogate decision making.

Family conferences challenge us because family members: (1) bring the complexity of their own relationships and interactions to the meeting, (2) have their own interests, (3) have individual emotional needs, (4) may have different preferences for information or decision-making, and (5) may disagree about the right course of action.

Family therapists tell us that families are more than a collection of individuals. Families are independent organisms with their own way of functioning. Some families talk things out calmly, some yell and scream, and others avoid conflict altogether. Family members also learn and assume their roles in the family. When these roles change out of necessity, others may not know how to react. For example, if before becoming ill, the matriarch was the family decision-maker, her daughter may feel insecure and anxious about making the monumental decision of withdrawing the matriarch's life support.

Creating a Neutral Discussion Zone

We don't expect you to become a family therapist. However, understanding family roles, relationships, and decision-making styles may help you navigate who to speak with when, who shouldn't be left out, and how to frame the issues.

CHALLENGE	COMMUNICATION TOOL
Family roles and decision-making preferences	Find out how the family makes decisions. Inquire about how the patient's illness may have changed these roles.
Family dynamics	Be curious without getting caught up in family history and pathology. Acknowledge different perspectives.

CHALLENGE	COMMUNICATION TOOL
A troublesome family member	Remain neutral and avoid taking sides or getting wrapped up in one person's perspective. Attend to the quiet family members or those who may have a "minority" opinion.
Divergent opinions	Name the disagreement. ("It sounds like you both agree on x, and you have different thoughts on y.")
Strong emotions	Acknowledge the various emotions in the room and respond with empathy.

Background questions that help you get to know the patient and how he or she functions within the family are especially useful. First, inquire about the patient, family roles, and relationships. For example, you could say, "Before we talk about these decisions, it would be helpful for me to hear more about your dad and his relationship with all of you." Subsequent questions can explore more about how the patient and family make decisions. For example, you might ask, "How has your dad (or your family) made decisions like these in the past? Is he the decision-maker or does he like to make sure that everyone has a voice?" Follow up with questions that deepen your understanding of the specifics of the family's decision-making processes. Some useful questions include "How could your family best make a medical decision and feel good afterward?" or "Who needs to be involved and what should the process look like?" or "Do you have any worries about how your family will deal with what is going on?" While we realize that you do not always have the luxury of knowing the answers to these questions before the family conference, remember that a social worker, psychologist, or nurse might know the answers and thus involve them in the family meeting.

To create a safe zone amidst the family dynamics, remain neutral in family interactions. Recognize the different family members equally so as not to ally yourself with one person or one side of the family. It may be hard to do this, particularly if you feel that one family member is being unfair, or even cruel. The family dynamics, however, predate the patient's illness and reflect lifelong patterns of interaction. You will not be able to change these patterns in a single brief conference, and if you try to change them, you're setting yourself up for failure. Instead, if there is a lot of tension or everyone starts fighting, it can be helpful to name the challenge and refocus the conversation on the patient. You might say, "I can see that there is a lot of tension here, and I think we can agree that we won't be able to resolve that today. I wonder if we could set that aside for now and focus on what's going on with your mother." The principle is that you are there to facilitate discussions focused on the patient's values, not to help manage longstanding family conflicts.

When it comes to caregiving, you should take a secondary role. The family has its own way for dealing with stress and you are an outsider. Let family members care for each other before you jump in. If one of the children begins to sob uncontrollably, it's better for her spouse or sister to hold her than for you to step in and assume that role. (This is just another example of the above principle of respecting the previously established family dynamics.) When you see constructive displays of empathy from family members to each other, acknowledge and reward them. If, however, the family members are not caring for each other, you should step in with empathy. Besides helping to respond to some-one's emotions, there may be value for the family to see you model empathy.

RESPONDING TO EMOTIONS WITH WORDS: FAMILY STYLE	
Jorge (son): *"We can't lose mom. We have to do everything."* Lucia (daughter): *"Jorge – I just can't watch her suffer like this."*	
Unifying empathic statements, following the NURSE framework:	
Name the emotions – everyone's.	"Jorge, it seems like it was shocking to arrive today and see your mom so ill. And, Lucia, you're understandably sad about what your mother has gone through."

Understand the emotions.	"I can't imagine how difficult it must be to see your mom go through all of this and still be so sick."
Respect (praise) the family. Name the shared interest – the patient!	"It's wonderful to see how you both advocate for your mom."
Support the patient and family.	"Our team will be here for your mom and your family as you all go through this."
Explore the emotions.	"Can each of you tell me a little more about what you're most worried about?"

When Families Need to Decide for a Patient

When patients are unable to participate, family members are ethically and legally empowered to serve as the surrogate decision-maker. Clinicians may therefore need to talk to families about medical choices, and we have noticed some common pitfalls in these conversations. Perhaps most problematic is when clinicians ask family members to decide on life-sustaining treatments for a patient, rather than asking them to assess what their loved one would choose in the given situation. This is a subtle but important difference. In making decisions for the patient, family members often confront their own hopes and fears about the patient's illness and death, and if the question about preferences is not anchored specifically to the patient, the family may become even more anxious. We recommend asking the family to represent what the patient would say: "If your mother was sitting in a chair with us, what would she say about this?" One study indicates that this question yields more accurate answers and, in our experience, asking what the patient would say lifts a bit of the responsibility and guilt from the family's shoulders.

Also, keep in mind that many families need help identifying and sorting through the patient's values (some of which may conflict) as they try to apply them to the medical decisions at hand. This is particularly true when applying large constructs ("He loves playing with his grand-children") to specific decisions about treatments and how they may impact the patient's longevity, function, and quality of life. Questions like, "If your mom could hear what we are saying, what would be most important to her?" or "As your dad was getting sicker, what did he worry about the most?" can shine a light on the patient's values and priorities and help you better understand the patient as a person. We similarly recommend avoiding phrasing that asks what the patient or family "wants," as it can lead to aspirational answers and may give the false impression that choices exist (about living or dying, for example). Of course families *want* their loved one to get better! Instead, by asking what the patient would *say* or *do*, you can keep the conversation grounded in what is happening now.

PITFALL	COMMUNICATION TOOL
Asking the family to decide for a patient. ("What do *you* want us to do?")	Ask the family what the patient would *say* ("If she could talk with us right now, what would she tell us to do?") or *think* ("What would your father think about his quality of life if he was dependent on a mechanical ventilator long term?")
Focusing on a single legal decision-maker. ("You're the proxy, we follow what you say.")	Respect other decision-making models. ("How does your family usually make decisions like this?")
Overlooking stresses of caregiving. ("I don't know if you've been here at the hospital.")	Explore stresses and identify support services. ("How are *you* coping?")

The second pitfall is rigidly focusing on a single, legal, surrogate decision-maker. Despite legal documents and state laws that designate order of surrogates, all families approach decision-making differently. For example, many families prefer to make decisions for their loved one collaboratively or even by consensus. Thus, even if the husband is the legal surrogate, the clinician typically meets with the entire family about what is going on with the patient. And while the husband may make the "final decision," he often wants to get the family's opinion and, if possible, agreement. Clinicians can help by engaging all key family stakeholders and honoring unofficial roles with statements like, "I can see that all of you feel deeply about what happens." Chances are the "official" decision-maker will feel some relief at knowing that the family has been able to come together on important decisions. We recommend that clinicians begin by asking how the family wants to make the decision and honor their preference if possible.

The third pitfall occurs when clinicians overlook the stress of caregiving. Family members in these scenarios are always stressed, sometimes anxious, and occasionally depressed. In one large study of patients with life-threatening diseases, 40% of families spent all of their savings caring for the patient. In addition to this huge financial burden, family members who have experienced the life-threatening illness of a loved one are at risk for posttraumatic stress disorder, and this risk rises with the length and complexity of the illness. The rate of posttraumatic stress disorder is even higher for family members who have had to make medical decisions for their loved one at the end of life. Think of the family as stressed individuals who will function better if supported. Ask them how they are doing and what you can do to help them get through their loved one's illness. Often the family has simple problems that you can refer to the social worker (e.g., help with a letter to their boss, or paying for parking). Families are very appreciative of your small efforts to help them and view these as evidence of your trustworthiness.

Similar to your interactions with individual patients, empathizing with family members' emotions is critical to creating a neutral zone for productive communication. In our experience running family meetings, the most common emotions we see are guilt and grief. Families feel guilty about "pulling the plug" on a loved one. You can address this by asking for the patient's view and allowing some time and space for the anticipatory grief they will experience as death approaches. Sometimes grief is not so much the issue as worry that they are abandoning the patient. After all, your family is supposed to take care of you! Of course, that means different things in different families, cultures, and religious traditions, so clinicians need to look to the family for guidance. For example, many patients and families in the US value intervention (doing something is better than doing nothing) and autonomy. Thus, the default decision for many families in the US is to do everything possible to improve their loved one's health.

Making a recommendation to the family that is grounded in the patient's values can go a long way in removing a burden from the family. The language you use here is important: lead with the things you *will* do and offer care you think will best help the patient in ways meaningful to them. Asking the family if they want to be "aggressive" or do "everything" implies that choices focused on comfort or palliation are "giving up." Similarly, talking about "withdrawing care" or "stopping life support" may heighten worries that the family is abandoning the patient. The recommendation might look like, "I suggest we use all medications and treatments that add to his comfort and stop anything that interferes with that goal. Would you like to hear more about what that might look like?"

Clinical Teams Also Have Their Own Dynamics

Many family meetings in the hospital involve multiple health care providers – the primary nurse, the social worker, the critical care clinicians, and members from the primary team. Clinicians should approach the family as a team that shares the common goal of supporting the family and providing the best care to the patient. Sports teams only achieve high functional standards with frequent deliberate practice. Medical teams differ from sport teams in that medical teams often include a number of individuals from different disciplines thrown together for a single event with success measured by the quality of care provided.

Many of these barriers to effective care team performance can be addressed by learning from the structured approach used by high-functioning sports teams or, in the hospital setting, resuscitation teams. A basketball team might prepare for a big game with warmup drills; a code team leader establishes situational awareness by briefly summarizing the case. Similarly, the care team ought to conduct a pre-meeting to prepare each participant for their role and ensure all clinicians are functioning as one team.

A high-functioning team creates an atmosphere of psychological safety for team members to express their views. The team leader's role includes creating the opportunity for team members to share opinions and arrive at a consensus by using empathic supportive phrases toward team members and giving all voices the space to contribute.

After the family conference, team members can debrief on what went well and describe areas for improvement in the future. These deliberate reflections encourage team members to identify specific learning points they can then incorporate into future practice.

Roadmap: Conducting a Family Conference

Notice that this roadmap has many parallels to the roadmaps for talking about serious news (GUIDE, Chapter 3) and discussing late-stage goals of care (REMAP, Chapter 8). Those fundamentals apply to family conferences, but here we also focus on the group dynamics that accompany such meetings.

1. ***Pre-meet*** *and prepare for who's going to be invited and the messages you hope to share.* In general, all family members who want to be present should be able to attend. The only exception would be if a patient with decision-making capacity indicated that certain people should not be included. Inviting some family members but not others can be seen as taking sides and may decrease one's ability to be an impartial patient advocate.

    Before sitting down with the family, participating health care providers should meet together to get on the same page medically, share information about the family, and agree on key points. This will enable you to deliver a clear and consistent message that will not be undercut by another provider.

It also allows clinicians to decide who will facilitate the meeting and what everyone present will contribute. The group should also crowdsource a headline to make sure that all clinicians are on the same page regarding the key information to provide the family. Do not skip this step! It is essential for minimizing confusion and conflict. Finally, securing a room with some privacy enables everyone involved to speak more freely.

2. ***Introduce*** *all participants and the purposes of the conference.* If you are facilitating, ask the other clinicians to give their names and roles in caring for the patient; ask family members to state their relationship and caregiving responsibilities. The facilitator might outline the purpose by saying, "I want to tell you how your dad is doing medically. I also want to make sure that you understand what we are doing for him and what we're watching for. Finally, we want to learn from you his values and goals so that we can make decisions that are the ones he would make if he could be with us right now. Are there any other things you want to make sure we discuss?" Families often respond to this question with a list of specific questions about what is happening or will happen. We suggest that, rather than jumping right in and answering these questions, you first acknowledge their importance ("Those are great questions, let me write them down") and try to assess what the family knows before trying to answer them ("I will make sure I answer your questions. I wonder if, first, you could tell me what other people are telling you about what is going on with your mom?").

3. ***Assess*** *what the family knows and* ***attend*** *to different perspectives.* Ask the family what they've been told about the patient's illness, and what they have observed. This enables you to assess how well they understand the medical situation, how they are doing emotionally, and how you should frame your summary of the clinical condition. If a family says, "We think he is dying," it is likely to lead to a very different conversation than if they say, "The doctors say he is not likely to get better, but we are praying that he gets better. He is such a fighter." Notice the emotion data in what the family says. Ask them if they want detailed information and whether they find statistical information helpful. Attend to the various perspectives, emotions, and information needs in the room. And make sure to pay attention to particularly quiet family members or those who seems to have a minority opinion. Including their input earlier will keep the conversation from getting derailed later.

4. ***Update*** *the family. Describe the clinical situation, and address questions and concerns.* Begin by asking permission to share your view. Start with the "big picture" or "headline," as described in Chapter 3. While you may want to name specific parameters that are being monitored, skip detailed pathophysiology. Give important information in small chunks, pausing intermittently to make sure they understand and to let them ask questions. The entire overview should take no more than a couple of minutes. If it takes longer, you have probably not prepared a clear enough message prior to the conference. Check for comprehension after you have finished by asking, "Does my explanation make sense? Is there anything that is not clear?" After providing information, it is important to ask explicitly for questions and concerns. Different family members may have different concerns. If possible, we ask, "What other questions or concerns do you all have?" until there are no more questions. If one person seems to dominate, invite other family members to speak. ("Can I see if any other family members have questions?")

5. ***Empathize*** *with the patient and family, attending to the various emotions in the room* (see "Responding to emotions with words: Family style," above). When people understand the medical information they've been told, particularly if it is serious, it is normal for them to react emotionally. Acknowledge the affective content of the family's concerns and questions and respond to their emotion explicitly (see "Responding to Emotions with Words" in Chapter 3), resisting the temptation to pile on more medical information. Responding to emotions helps people feel understood and allows them to process information. Try to acknowledge the emotions of all family members, ideally in a way that unifies the family and finds common ground. For example, statements such as, "It's clear that you both want what's best for your mom" or "I know there is a difference of opinion here, and it's also obvious that you both love your father very much" can highlight shared values and keep the patient at the center. Finally, it may help to ask if there is anything you can do to help the family members themselves. ("What can we do to help you to get through this difficult time?")

6. ***Prioritize*** *the patient's values and discuss how they should influence decision-making.* As noted earlier, focus on what the patient would prioritize, say or think (e.g., "If your dad was sitting here and could hear what we are saying, what would he say?"). Some family members find this question difficult

to answer; particularly when the patient's wishes conflict with what they would want for themselves. For example, a daughter might say, "My dad would never have wanted to live like this, but I don't want you to stop." While she is telling you that her dad would not want treatment focused on existence with this quality of life, she is also telling you that she feels guilty over being asked to make a life-and-death decision. Acknowledge the surrogate's perspective and remind her that her role is to tell you what her dad would want. You might say, "I hear how important your dad is to you and that you don't want to lose him. And I appreciate you telling me what your dad would say, so we can respect his values." Often, such a statement will lead to a discussion of the daughter's guilt and conflict, which may then lead her to let go of her own agenda and honor her father's.

7. **Align** *with the patient's values and support the family.* Use reflective summary statements to ensure that you have understood their values accurately (e.g., "As I listen, it sounds like your dad's independence is what is most important to him and that he wouldn't want his life prolonged if we didn't think we could get him back home again. Do I have that right?"). This helps them feel heard and understood, and it can even help family members understand each other better. Use your shared understanding of the patient's values to align the medical care with those values. We think clinicians in these conferences should make clear recommendations based on the patient's values. Begin by asking permission to offer a recommendation, and then propose a plan that honors the patient's goals. After that, you may want to talk about the therapies that don't match this approach. Share the "airtime" by explicitly asking for the family's thoughts. Remember – always start with what you *will* do to care for patients in a way that supports their values. Starting with a long list of therapies you want to withhold can feel to the family like abandonment.

8. **Summarize** *the messages that you want the family to take away from the meeting and provide a concrete follow-up plan.* If the discussion focused on goals of care, the summary should focus both on consensus decisions and on areas of disagreement. Be realistic about outcomes and timeframes. Recognize that families may need more time for processing before deciding and think carefully about what decisions truly need to be made urgently and those that can wait ("This is a lot to process. How about if we give you some time to think together, and we can meet again later in the week").

In addition, talk about milestones that may affect future decision-making. For example, if you decide upon a trial of antibiotics, then talk about what criteria will be used to know whether the antibiotics are working. Finally, specify the next time you will talk to someone in the family ("I'll give an update to whoever is here for rounds tomorrow"), so they have some sense of continuity.

One more thing: We define a successful family meeting as one in which the family leaves feeling heard and cared for, and the clinician identifies a treatment plan that aligns with values. That said, people cannot always come to agreement. We'll talk more about how to handle conflict in Chapter 10. In the meantime, remember that after about an hour of talk, no more good is likely to come out of the family meeting. If the meeting is stalling out, take a break or end the meeting and come back another time.

VALUE SKILLS

The acronym "VALUE" was coined by J. Randall Curtis, and encompasses all of the skills outlined in this chapter. In a large ICU study, VALUE was part of an intervention that improved family satisfaction and decreased their distress. The acronym stands for: Valuing and appreciating what the family said ("I really appreciate your coming to the meeting today," "Your help in telling us about your brother's values is really important in enabling us to develop the best plan"); Acknowledging the family's emotions ("I imagine that this is not what you wanted to hear"); Listening and Understanding the patient as a person ("Tell me what your Dad enjoyed before all this happened," "What would your dad think of all this?"); and Eliciting questions ("What concerns do you have?").

A Challenging Moment in a Family Conference

This exchange picks up in the middle of step 4 of the roadmap, with the physician checking in for family members' concerns. He is speaking with the patient's wife Kim and their son Jaylen.

WHAT HAPPENED	WHAT WE CAN LEARN
Dr. A: Given the medical situation I have just described, what concerns you most?	*Eliciting family concerns.*
Kim (wife): I'm just worried about whether he is going to make it.	*Notice the invitation to discuss death.*
Jaylen (son): We have to think positive. He *is* going to make it, isn't he, Doc?	
Dr. A: It sounds like each of you deals with the uncertainty in different ways.	*Notes that family members have different reactions and does not support one viewpoint at the expense of the other, which would be taking sides.*
Jaylen: That's certainly true.	
Dr. A: It's also clear to me that you both love him very much. He's fortunate to have you both as advocates.	*Unifying empathic statement that underscores their shared value – love and care of the patient.*
Kim: We do. [Jaylen nods agreement and smiles at his mother]	
Dr. A: Could you tell me what you think your husband and dad, Matthew, would say if he were sitting here?	*Eliciting the patient's values using specific instructions to the family.*
Kim: I think he would say that if he could only be alive like this, he wouldn't want it.	
Dr. A: [to Kim] Okay. [to Jaylen] What do you think?	*Inviting each family member to participate.*
Jaylen: He would probably want to be like this only if he had a chance to survive.	

WHAT HAPPENED	WHAT WE CAN LEARN
Dr. A: Do you mean, if he had a chance to survive and improve enough to get off the breathing machine?	*Asking a clarifying question.*
Jaylen: Yes. He's a fighter though.	
Dr. A: [looking at Kim, then Matthew] I appreciate you both sharing that with me, particularly since I haven't had the chance to talk to him myself. [To Jaylen] It sounds like you know him as a fighter, and that you want to help fight for him.	*Expressing gratitude and reaffirming the importance of the family's role in the decision process.*
Jaylen That's absolutely right!	
Dr. A: Could I suggest some things that you could do to help him?	*Deciding not to confront the son, but rather to form an alliance first.*
Jaylen: Yes.	
Dr. A: I think it would be very comforting for him for you to spend a little time talking to him each day – put your hand on his and tell him about your day. You could also tell him about your daughter. You can even tell him your version of what the doctors think. That kind of touch and talk are enormously soothing, and he could only get that from you.	*Identifying strategies to enable the family to be present with the patient.*
Later ...	
Dr. A: I think I understand better now about Matthew's views and values, and also about your concerns. Could I now talk about what I think would be the next best step medically, and get some input from you both?	*Signposting a new direction in the conversation and asking permission to proceed.*

Essential skills for managing family dynamics	Helpful Phrases
Stay neutral in family conflict. Table interpersonal conflicts to focus on the patient.	"I can see that there is a lot of tension here that we won't be able to resolve today. I wonder if we could set that aside for now and focus on what is going on with your mom."
Assess how the family prefers to make decisions.	"How has your family made decisions like this in the past?"
Find common ground. Focus on the patient as the shared interest.	"I can see how much you both love your mom."
When there is a difference in opinion, name the dilemma using reflective summary statements.	"One the one hand, I hear you, Lucia, saying x, and on the other hand, Jorge, I hear you saying y … " "It sounds like you both agree on x, and you have different thoughts on y."
Attend to the quiet ones.	"I'd like to hear from all of you if I can. Do any of the rest of you have something you'd like to add?" "Mrs. Y, I'd love to hear your thoughts on all of this."
Be realistic about outcomes and timeframes. Recognize that the family may need more time before coming to a decision.	"This is a lot to process, and we don't need to make any decisions today. Why don't you take some time to talk things over together, and I'll check in again tomorrow."
Remember that almost nothing good comes out of a family meeting after an hour of talk. If the meeting is stalling out, take a break or end the meeting and come back another time.	"We've talked through a lot today, and I thank you all for your time. How about if we all take some time to process this and regroup to talk more another day?"

The Bottom Line

Remember that each family member needs your individual attention, and also that the individuals in a family collaborate to form a unit with a life of its own (which you should observe and not interfere with).

RECOGNIZING WHAT A FATHER GAVE TO A SON

I was asked to talk to the family of a patient who had been in the MICU for nine months. This family, I was told, was very resistant and kept saying that they wanted "everything" done; I asked the two sons, "What do you think your dad would want if he was sitting here and could hear what everyone was saying about his illness?" One son immediately said, "He would never want this. He was very clear that if he could not go fishing and be active, that this would be a horrible existence." The other son piped in; "But we can't tell you not to do something that might help him. He was always there for us." Knowing this, I was able to acknowledge how much they cared for their dad and that they had done everything that might help him. What they needed to do now, I suggested, was to attend to their father's wishes. Rather than asking what surrogate decision-makers "want," this story reminds me that I need to orient surrogates to their role – which is helping me to understand the patient.

Maximizing Your Learning

This chapter contains many complex skills to potentially practice. One advantage of working on family conference skills is that often there is another clinician present who can give you feedback. If you have a chance, speak to the clinician before the conference and prepare that person to give you feedback. Tell them you are trying to improve your communication and ask them if they could give you a couple of minutes of feedback after the conference. Tell them the skill you are trying to practice and what you want them to look for. Finally, tell them that you find the most helpful feedback to be descriptive – what did you say and how did the other person respond?

Further Reading

Curtis, J. R., and D. B. White, Practical guidance for evidence-based ICU family conferences. *Chest*, 2008, **134**(4): 835–43.

Goold, S. D., B. Williams, and R. M. Arnold, Conflicts regarding decisions to limit treatment: A differential diagnosis. *JAMA*, 2000, **283**(7): 909–14.

Hammond, S. A., *Thin Book of Appreciative Inquiry*, 3rd ed. Thin Book Publishing Company, Bend, Oregon, 2013.

Lautrette, A., M. Darmon, B. Megarbane, et al., A communication strategy and brochure for relatives of patients dying in the ICU. *N Engl J Med*, 2007, **356**(5): 469–78.

McDonagh, J. R., T. B. Elliott, R. A. Engelberg, et al., Family satisfaction with family conferences about end-of-life care in the intensive care unit: Increased proportion of family speech is associated with increased satisfaction. *Crit Care Med*, 2004, **32**(7): 1484–8.

October, T. W., J. O. Schell, and R. M. Arnold, There is no I in team: Building health care teams for goals of care conversations. *J Palliat Med*, 2020, **23**(8): 1002–03.

Schenker, Y., M. Crowley-Matoka, D. Dohan, G. A. Tiver, R. M. Arnold, and D. B. White, I don't want to be the one saying "we should just let him die": Intrapersonal tensions experienced by surrogate decision-makers in the ICU. *J Gen Intern Med*, 2012, **27**(12):1657–65.

Scheunemann, L. P., R. M. Arnold, and D. B. White, The facilitated values history: Helping surrogates make authentic decisions for incapacitated patients with advanced illness. *Am J Respir Crit Care Med*, 2012, **186**(6): 480–86.

Wendler, D. and A. Rid, Systematic review: The effect on surrogates of making treatment decisions for others. *Ann Intern Med*, 2011, **154**: 336–46.

10

• • • • • • •

Dealing with Conflicts between Clinicians and Patients

Moving from "Who's Right?" to "What's Our Shared Interest?"

Up to this point, we have talked about communication as a means of educating, supporting, and empowering patients and families, with the underlying assumption that, beneath it all, clinicians and patients can agree on the next step. But, what do we do when the clinician and patient don't agree? Consider the patient with metastatic colon cancer progressing despite fourth-line chemotherapy who wants you to try another treatment regimen – one you think won't help and may even make things worse. Or, consider the family members in the ICU who know their loved one is dying but insist on continuing all life-prolonging measures, even keeping the patient full code, when all you see is a patient who is suffering while he is dying. Or the more common disagreements over using nontraditional medicines to treat COVID, or even fights over whether the patient has COVID.

These are uncomfortable situations for most clinicians. The term "conflict" may seem excessive for many disagreements, but clinicians often back off at the smallest sign of conflict. Most of us just don't like to argue. Plus, we consider the notion of supporting and comforting the patient and family as central to our mission, and it can be unsettling when we are not aligned. Sometimes we even assume that disagreement means our expertise is being called into question, and that makes us react either by saying, "I can't do that," or by withdrawing and deferring to "whatever the patient wants." Neither of these two reactions allows us to discuss our differences of opinion, explore the options, and come up with an agreed-upon plan with which we can all live.

How do better communication skills help address a conflict? They do so by shifting the focus from "Who's right?" to "What's our shared interest?" In complex medical situations, the different participants – physicians, nurses, other clinicians, patients, and family members – all need to contribute, and their different perspectives and insights will not necessarily all point in the same direction. Clinicians usually assume that conflict is undesirable and destructive. And certainly that can be true when conflict is handled poorly and the resulting bad feelings overwhelm the discussion. However, conflict handled well can be productive and enhance relationships, and the clarity that results can lead to improved decision making.

In this chapter, we focus on conflicts between clinicians and patients (or families). We'll tackle how to approach conflicts with colleagues in Chapter 11. That said, we know that conflicts with patients and colleagues can feel interlinked when they involve patient care, and we'll break down strategies for each.

How to Recognize When Conflict Exists

We often fail to notice that a conflict is unfolding, or that it's serious, until very late. By then, frustration can lead us to say something that we later regret. The earlier you can detect that another person doesn't agree with you, the earlier you can shift your approach. A variety of clues can help you recognize a conflict before things get out of hand. One such clue occurs when you begin to feel that you're talking in circles and the conversation is going nowhere. Another is when you make internal negative judgments about the other person – they're "not getting it," "clueless," or "in denial" – and, as a result, you feel angry or frustrated. A further clue is when you find yourself feeling fed up and wanting to shrug your shoulders and say "Whatever," just to be able to withdraw from the situation. When we see these signals, we know we are about to get stuck in an unproductive place. At that moment, it is probably best to (1) stop what you are doing (it's probably not helping anyway) and (2) avoid saying the first thing that comes to mind (which may make you feel better in the moment but will probably only make things worse).

What Helps You Handle Conflict?

Conflict requires you to step back from your instinctive reaction to educate, argue, or throw up your hands and move toward a nonjudgmental curiosity. Cultivating that nonjudgmental stance can be challenging, especially when you are trying to present your observations, expertise, and clinical judgment. This does not mean abandoning what you think is right; rather, it involves stopping for a minute and listening to the other person. Ask yourself: Why does this otherwise well-meaning person want something different in this situation than what I want? The "well-meaning" attribution is important. To deal with this successfully, you cannot afford to frame the other person as an idiot because people will pick up, perhaps from your nonverbal signals, that you're dissing them. You will not be successful if the other person feels dismissed. If you come across as arguing your point repeatedly (which we find ourselves doing when the other person "doesn't get it"), the other person will rapidly stop listening and may increase their arguments. They do this because they think that *you* "don't get it" and that you lack sufficient patience, courtesy, or respect to listen to what they have to say. So, instead, take a deep breath and summon your most patient self. If this sounds like it can take some time, consider the alternative. A full-blown conflict will consume far more time and energy than what we're suggesting.

A Roadmap to Dealing with Conflict

This roadmap is different from others in the book because the primary focus is on helping *you* find *your* path when you are at odds with someone (as opposed to helping someone else find their path). Don't misunderstand! You will still need to guide patients and families, but this chapter is about acknowledging that you can't do that successfully until you have found your own path, and that is an unfamiliar role for many clinicians. In a conflict, the only person you can change is yourself (although this may also leave space for the other person to change as well).

1. *Notice there is a disagreement.* When you feel conflict bubbling up, we suggest you take a proactive approach, rather than avoiding or minimizing the conflict. In this context, a conflict is a dispute, disagreement, or difference of opinion related to patient management, involving more than one individual, and requiring some decision or action. Thus, absence of shouting does not rule out conflict. You may notice repeated requests for the same thing, an edge of sarcasm, a bit of body language (e.g., subtle eye rolling or sideways glances). The cost of ignoring these more subtle gestures is that the real issue will be discussed when you are not around and without your input. You may notice that you feel irritated, bored ("this again?") or exasperated – your internal signals may be your most useful sensors for noticing conflict.

2. *Prepare your approach and start softly, finding a nonjudgmental entry point.* The key to intervening in a conflict is to raise the issue without attacking the other person or escalating the conflict. This requires empathy and perspective. You may need a minute to get ready (data from marital arguments show that this actually takes 20 minutes, so don't underestimate your irritability). You may find it valuable to ask yourself what we call "the humanizing question." *Why would a decent, rational, logical person want what they asked for (or do what they just did)?* The purpose of this question is twofold: you pause before rushing to judgment, and you create space for the other person to speak. Then restart the discussion by finding a starting point that names the topic in a descriptive and nonjudgmental way – instead of "I want to talk about your attitude," try "I feel like we're both talking

about what the best treatments would be. Could we start there?" Assuming you have the same goal, even if you may get to it in a different way, puts you on the same side.

3. *Invite the other person's perspective before you share yours, listening to and acknowledging their story, concerns, and needs.* Lead with curiosity. Turn your full attention to the other person and turn off your arguments for a few moments. If you are mentally preparing counterarguments, you are not really listening. Douglas Stone and colleagues describe three things to listen for: (1) their story of what has happened; (2) the emotions generated by what happened (theirs and yours); and (3) their view of their identity – how does it shape their views? This may also cause you to reflect on any identity triggers of your own that may be playing into the discussion (e.g., what does this say about me as a doctor?). Your goal here is not simply to mirror their words back to them; you need to provide them with evidence that you understand their view and their emotional reaction. For example, for some caregivers, talking about withholding any potentially life-prolonging treatments may threaten their sense of their caregiver role. (After all, wouldn't someone who loved the patient insist on doing whatever it took to help the patient survive?) If you can recognize that the caregiver in question is feeling an identity threat ("What kind of a wife would I be … ?"), you are more likely to interpret the caregiver's actions with compassion and provide the empathy needed to identify a shared path forward. (See Chapter 3 for suggestions about responding to emotions with words.)

4. *Identify what the conflict is about and try to articulate it as a shared interest.* At this point in the conversation, you can talk about your views and concerns. Be careful to withhold judgment by using language that focuses on the *problem* instead of on the *people*. Describe the issue in question in terms of a shared interest. This may require some reframing, and reframing topics from being emotionally charged to being a shared interest takes practice. For example, rather than telling a patient, "The treatment you found on the Internet won't help you," you might try, "I want to make sure you have access to the best treatments." A handy tip for reframing is to shift the focus from the person ("You're wrong") to the interest ("the best treatments").

5. *Brainstorm solutions that address the shared concern.* In conflicts between a clinician and patient, it is often the clinician's willingness to consider alternatives and talk about them that proves to the patient that the clinician

is willing to address their concerns. The key to talking about options is to list and explain what they are without saying which one is your first choice. Let the patient take them in and think about how each option meets the shared concern. One approach we find useful in situations where there is disagreement about whether a new treatment will be worthwhile is to offer a time-limited trial of a medical intervention. Note that this tactic of naming all the options need not conflict with the importance we placed earlier in the book on making a clear treatment recommendation grounded in the patient's values. It's just that when there is a conflict it can be useful to clearly demonstrate openness to the various treatment options available while helping the patient sort through how those options intersect with their various (and sometimes conflicting) values.

6. *Look for options that recognize the interests of everyone involved.* As a clinician, you routinely make judgments about the best medical care, and we routinely equate "best" with most effective. Negotiating productively might mean that you need to consider what would be "best" because it meets a patient's or family member's needs even though another option might be more biologically efficacious. There may also be options that you think are not reasonable. Coming to agreement on the action to take requires that you be clear for yourself about which options you can live with.

7. *Remember that not every conflict can be resolved.* In dealing with conflicts, a successful conversation is one that results in greater understanding on both sides. This does not mean that the conflict will be resolved, because, even using these principles, you will run into some conflicts for which there is just no easy way forward. In such a case, consider finding a third party that you both respect to moderate the discussion. An ethics consultant, someone from quality management (they often have people who mediate disputes) or a palliative care consult may help. Remember, conflicts occur because people care deeply about the issues and the people involved, which means that resolving the conflict will take time and effort. Two examples of non-resolvable conflicts may be requests for unproven COVID treatments (e.g., ivermectin) or for more opiates in situations where you are concerned about a substance use disorder. In both cases, you have tried to name shared values ("providing the best possible care"), listened to the patient's views, discussed numerous

pharmacological and nonpharmacological alternatives, and acknowledged the differing viewpoints. At some point, it is acceptable to say "I hear your view and I think we are going to need to agree to disagree. As a clinician, I cannot prescribe X in this situation." Continuing the discussion becomes counterproductive as it suggests that negotiation is possible and will likely lead to more frustration. Stressing that you want to care for the patient within those parameters is the best you can do.

When to drop the "but" and embrace the "and"

I was in a family meeting where a doctor kept saying, "We know you want your loved one to get better, but he's really, really sick." Afterward, the family complained that the doctors did not want their loved one to get better, that they did not feel the doctors were on their side. I remembered a conference where a speaker pointed out that the word "but" essentially discounts everything preceding it – it was an amazing revelation. In contrast, the word "and" allows two truths to stand side-by-side, even when they are in conflict. So, I reframed the issue by saying, "It sounds like the doctor says he is really sick and yet you still hope that he will get better." This worked much better. The family felt that I heard and understood them, which, in turn, made it easier for them to problem-solve around their loved one's illness.

Conversation Example, Demonstrating Roadmap

The following exchange, between Ms. J., a woman with advanced peritoneal carcinomatosis, and Dr. A. illustrates the roadmap.

WHAT HAPPENED	WHAT WE CAN LEARN
Ms. J: I've been thinking that I'd like to go to the hospital.	
Dr. A: Tell me what's been going on?	*Noting the disagreement internally, Dr. A makes a conscious effort to find a nonjudgmental starting point by exploring.*
Ms. J: I'm uncomfortable because of the fluid in my abdomen. I think I need an IV, because I can't eat – I feel too full.	

WHAT HAPPENED	WHAT WE CAN LEARN
Dr. A: It sounds like you're having a tough time.	*Listening to the patient's story about what's happened, using empathy to show that he understands the patient's viewpoint.*
Ms. J: Well, yes.	
Dr. A: I think we could do a better job with all these issues.	*Trying to articulate the shared interest: better symptom control.*
Ms. J: That's why I want to go to the hospital.	
Dr. A: Could you say why you are thinking about the hospital, versus outpatient treatments?	*Eliciting patient's reasoning.*
Ms. J: I think things will happen faster, that they will take care of me.	
Dr. A: It sounds like we need to focus on making you more comfortable. Could I make some recommendations at this point? I will talk about the pros and the cons of going to the hospital, okay?	*Asking permission to present options that meet the shared concern.*
Ms. J: Okay.	
Dr. A: If we did a bit more evaluation today, there are some medicines we could start now to make you more comfortable, so all of this could start sooner than having you go to the hospital. The pros of going to the hospital are that there are lots of nurses and doctors around to help you; the cons are that they would probably discharge you after only a day, and the hospital doctors would expect the rest of the treatment to happen at home.	*Presenting the option of outpatient intervention, also the option of inpatient intervention.*
Ms. J: What could we do right now?	

WHAT HAPPENED	WHAT WE CAN LEARN
Dr. A: Here is what I think …	*Having negotiated the conflict, Dr. A makes medical recommendations now that Ms. J is more receptive.*

When People Are Rude

When patients have been rude or uncivil you may feel quite justified treating them similarly. We are rarely overtly rude to patients in return, but we may be tempted to dismiss their concerns, talk over them, or distance ourselves – all of which count as being rude (as does sarcasm). Such is human nature. However, responding in such a way is likely to escalate the conflict. For most of us, opting for a more positive, resolution-oriented response requires some serious self-management skill. Again, looking at the emotion as data is helpful – their anger likely represents frustration, sadness, hurt, or fear – and figuring this out will help you know what to say next. The measure of your skill is the level of empathy you can bring to the situation.

On the other hand, you are not professionally obliged to be the object of demeaning or threatening statements. You do, however, need to explain yourself. If a patient or family member is screaming or abusive, it's okay to tell the person in a calm voice, "I realize you feel very strongly about this. I find it hard to talk to you when you are using that kind of language." (Notice that we did not say, "But I find it hard … " because the "but" can make the "feel very strongly" come across as a concession rather than a statement of understanding.) Many people in these situations are unaware of how they are coming across, and if you point this out, they will usually rein themselves in. On rare occasions, you may feel that someone is truly threatening; in that case, you should stand up, note your concern, leave the room, and call security. This framework will also work when a patient or family member makes an inappropriate comment based on gender, ethnicity, or other personal characteristics. Imagine a patient makes a sexist comment about your appearance. You might say "I am here as your doctor. When you make comments about my figure, I feel like you are not respecting my training and skills. Your comment makes it hard for me to care for you as a physician."

When the Conflict Seems Unresolvable

If you are having a tough time finding any mutually acceptable options, and the request from the patient, family, or colleague still stands, step back from the situation (and the frustration) for a moment. There are some conflicts that are rooted in different values that better communication will not resolve. For example, a patient and family who feel that life is precious regardless of the quality of the life may butt heads with a doctor who is strongly committed to quality of life. If this family conflicts with this doctor about continued mechanical ventilation for a patient who all agree is dying of sepsis, it is not likely that a negotiation approach like the one we described will resolve the conflict – the meaning of ventilation for the family (increased length of life) is too different from the meaning of ventilation for the doctor (unacceptable quality of life).

When the conflict appears to be at a standstill, we suggest you ask yourself three reflective questions: (1) How important is this to the other person's core beliefs/values? (2) How important is this to my own core beliefs/values? (3) How flexible can I be in this case without compromising an important value of my own? The challenge is to be flexible without compromising your own integrity. Over time, we have found our own responses in these situations have become increasingly flexible, more accepting of what patients feel is really important, and less attached to biomedical outcomes.

There will be times that you find yourself faced with a situation in which you and a patient or family member cannot agree even after discussion and negotiation. If you've followed our approach, the remaining disagreement is likely to be about core values for each of you, and a situation like this can't be resolved with better communication skills. In these cases, you need to get help, such as an ethics consultant, a palliative care consultant, a colleague who can serve as a facilitator, or a person in quality management who handles disputes. You may need to agree that the different interests cannot be reconciled. In these cases, the communication skill is to disagree gracefully, without backing down from your value but also without describing the other person's value in a pejorative way. For instance, a patient told us what happened when she asked her primary care provider for a prescription to hasten her death. The primary care physician, in response, explained that she could not do that because she would not be able to live with herself afterward. At the same time, the primary care physician fully acknowledged the patient's terrible situation and the legitimacy of the request. This graceful disagreement led to a clear understanding on the part of the patient and continuation of the relationship. The patient accepted that the physician had very different beliefs about this but felt heard and understood.

The Bottom Line

Instead of digging your heels in, look for a nonjudgmental starting point, lead with curiosity, and identify a shared interest you can articulate.

Maximizing Your Learning

Conflict with patients and families challenges us to grow and learn, but it can also feel antithetical to our calling as clinicians. After all, we want our interactions with patients to be therapeutic, and it feels bad when the patient is more distressed after a visit with us than when they came in. After one of these encounters, take some time to honor how challenging these situations are! Be kind to yourself and find a private place to decompress and sort through your thoughts and feelings:

- Try post-hoc to answer the humanizing question about why a well-meaning person is taking this position. What are the values that are likely underlying the patient's stance or action? Where do their values butt up against your values?

- Reflect on the things you did well in addressing the conflict and celebrate those.
- Commit to one thing you'll do differently the next time you face a similar challenge or conflict and hold yourself to it. Remember, these are opportunities for growth (however painful) so make the most of it!

Further Reading

Back, A. L. and R. M. Arnold, Dealing with conflict in caring for the seriously ill: "It was just out of the question." *JAMA*, 2005, **293**(11): 1374–81.

Dugan, D. O., Praying for miracles: Practical responses to requests for medically futile treatments in the ICU setting. *HEC Forum*, 1995, **7**(4): 228–42.

Kahn, M. C., Understanding and engaging the hostile patient. *Mayo Clin Proc*, 2007, **82**(12): 1532–4.

Philip, J., M. Gold, M. Schwarz, et al., Anger in palliative care: A clinical approach. *Intern Med J*, 2007, **37**(1): 49–55.

Sager, Z. and J. Childers, Navigating challenging conversations about nonmedical opioid use in the context of oncology. *Oncologist*, 2019, **24**(10): 1299–304.

Shankar, M., T. Albert, N. Yee, and M. Overland, Approaches for residents to address problematic patient behavior: Before, during, and after the clinical encounter. *J Grad Med Educ*, 2019, **11**(4): 371–4.

Stone, D., B. Patton, and S. Heen, *Difficult Conversations: How to Discuss What Matters Most*, 2nd ed. Penguin Books, New York, 2010.

11

· · · · · · ·

Working Through Conflicts with Colleagues

From "Being Right" to "Making Things Right"

Looking for Value in Differing Points of View

In the previous chapter, we discussed managing conflicts between clinicians and patients (or families). Here we address conflicts with our colleagues, building upon what we learned in the last chapter and highlighting some key differences in the approaches between the two.

What do we mean when we talk about a conflict with a colleague? We're referring to any time you feel vulnerable, your professional identity is threatened, your self-esteem is implicated, or the issues at stake are important and the outcome is uncertain. Consider the ICU team that insists on doing the exact opposite of everything you recommend for a patient. Or the colleague who appears to hate every idea you have and is continually talking over you at meetings. Or the administrator who just removed funding from a project you feel passionate about.

Conflicts with our colleagues can lead to some of the most stressful moments in our work. They can be time-consuming, divisive, and emotionally exhausting. And many of us find talking through conflicts with our colleagues unpleasant – even worthy of dread. So, what to do? Usually, we try to convince or persuade, and if that doesn't work, we argue, blame, or give up and walk away – none of which helps resolve the conflict. Even worse, when we do address the conflict directly, we risk doing it in a one-sided way that feels like us versus them and only makes the disagreement – and the bad feelings that go along with it – worse. None of these approaches allow us to sort through our different perspectives and ideas, explore potential solutions, or find a pathway forward that everyone can accept. Moreover, such an approach can harm the relationship, making future collaboration even more challenging.

Yet conflict handled well can be a game changer – improving outcomes and relationships and enhancing collaboration. What we describe below is an approach to managing conflict that shifts the focus from "being right" to "making things right," and we have seen it improve not only the situation at hand but, in many cases, the relationship as well. Having communication skills to navigate even the stickiest situation at work will allow you to approach these situations with more equanimity and confidence, making it much less likely that you'll panic or put your foot in your mouth. It also improves the chance that you will be able to resolve conflicts in a way that keeps everyone's ideas in the mix (including yours!) and come to a resolution that all can embrace.

How Do Conflicts with Other Clinicians Differ from Conflicts with Patients?

When working with patients and families, conflict is most often generated by powerful emotions such as frustration, disappointment, loss, grief, and fear, and these often possess undercurrents of powerlessness and shame. When we face conflicts with other clinicians, the powerful emotions are the same, but the social contract is different. What do we mean by this? With a patient, the professional relationship allows for emotions to be dealt with; managing emotion is part of a therapeutic relationship. On the other hand, with many professional colleagues, we don't assume that talking about our emotions is part of our professional work. (There are exceptions, but usually we clinicians talk about this stuff only with people we really trust.)

In addition, other clinicians – especially those from a different professional discipline – may have concerns about power and respect. Power influences how disagreements or conflicts are presented. A clinician who is higher on the power hierarchy (say, an attending physician) is often treated more respectfully than a clinician lower on the power hierarchy. Consequently, the clinician with less power (e.g., a nurse) is more likely to be tentative in raising a disagreement, and the clinician with more power (e.g., the attending physician) is more likely to miss that the nurse is actually quite upset. The implication is that the higher you are on the power hierarchy, the more attuned you need to be to concerns of other clinicians. If you are casual in handling an issue important to others, you risk having them feel that their work is not respected. In fact, we would take this further and suggest that the person with more power has a responsibility to make it psychologically safe for those with less power to disagree with them.

Thus, when working through a conflict with a colleague, the question ought to be: How do I show that I'm really interested in hearing their views, and what do I need to do to earn enough trust so that they tell me? This requires establishing a safe space with your colleague. As with patients, the conversation merits your full attention and should be held privately, out of earshot of patients and other colleagues. And, as with patients, you need to demonstrate openness and curiosity.

What if you're the one with less power in the relationship? This can be tricky. Individuals in this situation can also try to create a safe space, which can be surprisingly effective. The powerful person is more likely to make themselves vulnerable if their own security is not challenged. We encourage those with less power to "test the water" and see if the more powerful person is able to hear you. Do they respond in a way that allows a further conversation? If not, the situation may need to be escalated to one's superiors who can help address the conflict.

The issue of how to address your colleagues' emotions is also tricky. While we have advocated attention to emotion and empathy for patients and family members, our experience is that empathy for colleagues is sometimes misinterpreted as condescending. In particular, clinicians higher on the power hierarchy need to be careful about how they address the emotions of their colleagues. Many clinicians implicitly subscribe to a belief that their emotions should not be part of their work and that showing emotion represents weakness. Thus, clinicians need to respond carefully to their colleagues' emotions, framed in a way acceptable to the colleague. Often, you may be on safer ground talking about emotions generated by the situation (e.g., "This is a really sad situation") rather than your colleague's visible emotions (e.g., "I can see you are really upset"). We've referred to this as "third-person neutral empathy." And definitely stay far away from discussing emotion in a way that could be seen as pejorative (e.g., "You are personally involved with this patient, aren't you?"). As with patients, you may want to name emotion at a step lower than what you are observing (e.g., "I think anyone would be frustrated by what has happened") as a way of acknowledging the emotion in a way that is unlikely to be viewed as critical or condescending.

Creating a Neutral Discussion Zone: Working on Me First

Conflict is inescapable; it's how you handle it that matters. We suggest starting with the end in mind: you want to improve the relationship, circumstances, and outcomes. You are *not* trying to win, shame, or humiliate – that will only make things worse. Keeping your wish to improve the situation and relationship in mind during the conversation will help you maintain your balance and purpose – and help you avoid being hijacked by your emotions into attack mode. Try leading with something like, "I'm hoping this conversation will help us work together more effectively in the future." Naming that you are trying to make things better for both of you can help put the other person at ease. However, to make good on this commitment, you must be able to walk the talk.

How do you do this? By being ready and willing to grow and learn yourself. Stone and colleagues call this creating a "learning conversation," in which you take deliberate steps to understand the breadth of the problem, including not only learning about the other person's perspective but also about your role in the conflict. This can be painful, because chances are that you'll learn some things about how you are perceived or the impact of your actions that you weren't aware of before. With this in mind, we offer some caution. If you aren't ready to learn about yourself (or are primarily focused on making the other person see how wrong they are), stop and take a step back. You aren't yet ready to have a learning conversation. However, if you are prepared for and open to the feedback that comes in return (the "tuition" we pay), these conversations can help you grow and learn in remarkable ways, even as you improve the working relationship with the other person.

As with all treacherous journeys, we recommend starting at the beginning, which, in this case, means working on yourself – and your own interpretation of events – first. Stone and colleagues call this step "mastering your stories," and we believe this pre-work is essential for navigating conflict effectively. To do so, you think long and hard about the events, how you feel about them, what they mean to you (or say about you), and how you are interpreting them *before* you talk to the other person.

To master your stories, we recommend that you ask yourself four questions. The first question is the "humanizing question" you learned about in Chapter 10: "Why is this otherwise well-meaning person behaving in this challenging way?" This helps you find the kindest possible explanation for the other person's behavior, including assuming good intentions, which keeps you calm and makes space for curiosity and empathy. After all, when it comes down to it, it is our interpretation of another person's behavior (and the negative intentions we assume explain the behavior) that makes us upset, angry, or frustrated. Take for example, the person who cuts you off while driving. You might assume that they are thoughtless and careless – a hazard on the road! – until you learn that they were racing to the hospital where their son was just brought by ambulance. Sometimes, we need help finding a kind interpretation of the other person's behavior. In that case, phone a friend you trust for their insight. Often, someone who doesn't have skin in the game has the perspective needed to interpret the other person's behavior with compassion.

The next three questions to ask yourself are the same three questions we want you to listen for when you hear the other person's perspective. Only this time, we ask you to listen to yourself to get a handle on your own thoughts and feelings. The three questions are:

(1) What happened? The point is, your story of the event most likely differs from their story of the event.

(2) What are the feelings here (yours and theirs)? Stone and colleagues recommend that we get all our feelings out on the table privately and then *negotiate* with them. For example, in negotiating with your feelings, you may realize that the anger you are experiencing has less to do with the other person's behavior and more to do with your own sense of shame at not having done something in a way that met your own expectations.

(3) What identity concerns does this conflict bring up for me? What might this conflict say about me (as a nurse, a doctor, a colleague, a parent)? What identity threats might the other person be feeling?

Managing conflict with someone you work with or care about requires a great deal of personal insight, and doing this soul searching gives you a better sense of your own role in the conflict. It also grounds you when you face feedback or information you might otherwise find threatening or destabilizing. For example, if you've thought long and hard about what identity triggers this conflict brings up for you, you'll find staying calm much easier if these triggers arise when you are navigating the conflict with the other person. All this pre-work also gives you a chance to reflect on what you are hoping to achieve by addressing the conflict as well as what may (or may not) be possible.

One final note. Earlier we said that, in conversations about conflict, the measure of your skill is the level of empathy you can bring to the situation. Sure, we meant for the other person, but we say it again here to remind you to extend your kindness and compassion to *yourself* as well. It is nearly impossible to interpret others kindly if you are unable to be kind to yourself. So, while we encourage you to be open to learning about your role in the conflict, we want you to do it as a caring friend to yourself. These situations are really hard, and all of us have bad days from time to time or handle things imperfectly. Give yourself credit for having the courage it takes to address conflict and embrace the personal growth that comes along with it.

Roadmap: Approaching Conflict with a Colleague

In navigating conflicts, the primary focus is on helping *you* find *your* path when you are at odds with someone. This means that you are first and foremost negotiating with yourself and only secondarily helping other people involved negotiate with themselves. This takes time and effort and can be uncomfortable – but it is less time-consuming and uncomfortable than letting a problem fester. There is deliberate over-lap between this roadmap and the one in Chapter 10, but there are subtle differences in approach as well.

1. ***Notice*** *when conflict is bubbling up.* The first step in managing a conflict effectively always involves recognizing that it is happening – the earlier the better – and taking a proactive role. The clues that conflict exists are similar whether the conflict is with a colleague, a patient, or a friend: circular conversations; closed or hostile body language; criticism; internal feelings of unease, threat, or frustration; and a tendency to want to avoid that person. When that happens, take notice, then mentally "step back" and pause. Remember, absence of yelling does not mean you are in a conflict-free zone, and if you are feeling the tension, chances are the other person is too.

2. ***Prepare*** *your approach instead of jumping in reactively.* To manage conflict well, you need to raise the issues in a way that avoids attacking the other person or inadvertently escalating the conflict. So, slow down before you respond! Being mindful and tapping into slow thinking improves your executive control. Then, look for the kindest possible explanation of the other person's behavior, assuming good intentions. As described earlier, it helps to ask yourself the "humanizing question": "Why is this otherwise well-meaning person behaving in this challenging way?" Remember the

"well-meaning" part is essential – you need to hold your colleagues in high positive regard to do this well – or your body language or word choice will betray you. Chances are this conflict exists because you both feel passionately and have good intentions – you just don't agree.

Does this mean we give everyone a pass on bad behavior? No, of course not. But pausing to look for the kindest explanation helps us keep a clear head and approach the situation calmly. It also invites the other person to rise to the good intentions you are giving them credit for, instead of becoming defensive and entering attack mode.

3. **Start softly** *to avoid provoking defensiveness.* This requires finding a nonjudgmental starting point that both sides can buy into. We find it helpful to name the *topic* in a descriptive and nonjudgmental way, instead of talking about the *person.* Instead of, "You really dropped the ball with that patient!" try "I noticed the patient's code status wasn't changed after our conversation with him, which caused confusion when the rapid response team was called. Can you tell me more about what happened there?" Stone and colleagues refer to this as the "third story," which is the story a neutral third party might tell and a version of the story that both parties in conflict can buy into. The "third story" names a shared common purpose while capturing the differences in a nonblaming, nonjudgmental way (e.g., "I can see that we're both committed to this being a successful endeavor. It's also clear to me that we are not 100% on the same page about how members of the leadership team work together, which I feel plays out in a conflict around education. I'm hoping to hear more about your perspective and share mine, so that we're able to work together more effectively"). You can also start the conversation by stressing your joint mission. Agreeing on the outcome leads to talking about the way to get there and decreases perceptions that the disagreement is personal (e.g., "I wonder if we can talk about how we can help Mrs. Bynum feel better. It's a complicated situation and I want to make sure we're on the same page. What are you thinking?")

4. **Invite** *the other person's perspective before you share yours.* Turn your full attention to the other person, and lead with curiosity. Allowing the other person to share first helps you to learn more about their perspective, which helps you to diagnose the conflict. And it helps them feel safer because they know they'll get to say their piece, and they have some control over how the discussion starts. You can see that the sample of a "soft start"

described above in Step 3 ends with an invitation: "I'm hoping to hear more about your perspective and share mine, so that we are able to work together more effectively." Inviting them to speak first and naming the "end outcome" you are hoping for (in this case, to work together more effectively) offers the other person some assurance that you aren't looking to "catch them out" or railroad them. When you are listening to their perspective, give them your full attention and listen for the three things Stone and colleagues taught us: the other person's story of what happened, the emotions generated by what happened (theirs and yours), and what the conflict may mean to their sense of identity. As mentioned earlier, we also recommend you make peace with what this conflict means to your identity prior to embarking on the conversation. Being surprised by an identity threat is destabilizing and can make it harder to stay neutral. Demonstrate active listening to show them that you understand their view and feelings. Once they've shared their perspective, go ahead and share yours.

5. **Use neutral language** *to reframe emotionally charged issues.* Emotionally charged issues will come up, as will new points of disagreement. When that happens, try to use language that diffuses the conflict instead of inflaming it. Using descriptive language ("It seems like we are interpreting the data differently") instead of "evaluative" language ("You're wrong") makes the conflict more discussable and keeps tempers at bay. Similarly, framing questions in a way that demonstrates curiosity instead of challenge helps keep the peace. For example, "what" or "how" questions ("What are you hoping will happen if we proceed down that path?" or "How are you thinking about this?") sound more like exploration and curiosity, whereas "why" questions ("Why do you want to do that?") risk sounding like an attack.

   We know this is hard! Keeping things neutral requires a great deal of self-control, and, quite frankly, often involves allowing barbs to pass unaddressed. There is no guarantee that the person with whom you are in conflict has read this book or is as committed as you are to avoiding out-and-out war. That's okay. Either they will settle down when they see you won't take the bait, or you'll identify that resolving the conflict isn't on their priority list. Either way, it helps you proceed with more peace of mind.

6. **Express empathy** *toward the situation, not the person.* No matter how "businesslike" we want to be, these situations generate emotions – lots of them, for everyone involved. As always, emotions need to be addressed

to allow everyone to settle down and the conversation to move forward productively. As described above, you need to respond to your colleagues' emotion but in a way that's consistent with what is expected at work – empathy focused on the *situation* instead of on the *person* ("third-person neutral empathy"). Instead of, "I can see that you're really upset," try "These situations are really tough." It shows you understand how the other person might be feeling, without pointing any fingers or risking being interpreted as condescending.

7. ***Find a path forward*** *that addresses both parties' concerns, creating new options where needed.* Find your points of shared interest ("We are clearly both committed to helping this project go as well as possible") and invite a discussion about how you might reach that shared interest together (e.g., "Let's try to think creatively about how everyone's concerns can be addressed"). In this situation, brainstorming so that each of you builds on the other's ideas tends to lead to the most collaborative, mutually acceptable outcomes. If tensions are still high, first inviting the other person to start the problem-solving brainstorming with what they would see as the best outcome can be disarming. For example, you might say, "From your standpoint, what would be the best outcome going forward?"

A Challenging Discussion between Two Physicians

The following exchange between two physician colleagues who have a patient care disagreement illustrates the roadmap, starting at Step 3. Dr. R is a nocturnist who cared for one of Dr. L's longtime primary care patients overnight, changing the plan from what Dr. L and the family decided at the time of admission.

WHAT HAPPENED	WHAT WE CAN LEARN
Dr. L: Hi, Dr. R. I saw Mr. C and his family this morning, and I was wondering if we could talk about his care.	A neutral invitation to discuss the patient's care, giving Dr. R time to find his footing.

WHAT HAPPENED	WHAT WE CAN LEARN
Dr. R: Sure. What's up?	
Dr. L: Well, the family is a little confused about what happened overnight. We had all decided to focus on comfort care and last night he was awakened for a bunch of tests and got started on antibiotics. I want to make sure we're all on the same page so we can support the family. Can you tell me more about what happened?	Starts softly describing the facts in a neutral way that both parties can buy into (the "third story") while clearly naming the gap. Then, Dr. L invites Dr. R to share his views of what happened.
Dr. R: Well, he has pneumonia on x-ray, so I thought he'd be more comfortable if I gave him IV antibiotics. And he was really confused, so I got the head CT and the rest of the tests to see what we could do to help.	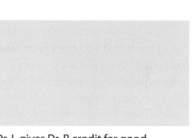
Dr. L: I saw all that, and I appreciate that you were trying to help Mr. C. My concern is that the family had decided they wanted to focus on comfort, and they specifically wanted to avoid tests and IVs because they agitate him. I wrote a goals of care note last night trying to summarize what we talked about.	Dr. L gives Dr. R credit for good intentions, highlighting their shared interest, which is taking good care of the patient. Then she follows by sharing her version of what happened.
Dr. R: I did, but I thought he deserved a chance to get better. I was just trying to take good care of the patient.	
Dr. L: I really do appreciate that you want to take good care of Mr. C, and I do too. His family also takes really good care of him, and they made a really hard and loving decision to focus on comfort, which they felt would be consistent with his wishes. So, they were upset and confused to see that the plan had changed, particularly because they weren't aware it was happening. I was	Dr. L underscores their shared interest – taking good care of the patient. Honoring this also helps avoid triggering identity threats in Dr. R, who truly believed he was working in the patient's best interest. Importantly, Dr. L also ignores the potential barb regarding what the patient "deserved," which prevents the conversation derailing.

WHAT HAPPENED	WHAT WE CAN LEARN
also confused, which probably seemed to them like you and I weren't working as a team.	Dr. L. then names her own emotions about the situation, deliberately naming them at a step lower than is likely true (in reality, she's pretty upset – and embarrassed that the patient was negatively impacted by team dysfunction).
Dr. R: Okay, I guess I can see that. Well, we can certainly shift to comfort now that we know what we are dealing with.	
Dr. L: Thank you, I think it's important that we do that. I also want to see if we can avoid situations like this in the future, because I think it's really hard on patients and families and makes our life harder.	Offers appreciation for remedying the immediate situation. Then begins dialogue about how they can work together better in future.
Dr. R: It might be, but it's impossible for us to know what every family wants and needs when they come in the middle of the night. For all I knew, they'd be upset if I didn't do all that stuff, so I figured it was better to err on the side of doing it. I know I would be upset if the admitting doctor didn't do everything they could for my dad.	
Dr. L: These situations are really tough.	Responding with empathy for the *situation* instead of the *person* shows Dr. R that Dr. L understands his feelings while minimizing the risk that Dr. R will perceive Dr. L as condescending.
Dr. R: They are!	

WHAT HAPPENED	WHAT WE CAN LEARN
Dr. L: So, it sounds like it's hard to balance what every individual needs in the middle of the night. It also sounds like there was some tension for you about not trying to reverse the acute condition, even though when I spoke with the family they were clear in their wishes for comfort care. Do I have that right?	Dr. L reflects back to Dr. R's statements to show she understands. She also clearly names the gap (that the family was clear about their wishes) being careful to avoid using any language that might imply judgment.
Dr. R: I guess so. [pauses for several seconds] You're right, though, the family was clear about their wishes. [pauses] I guess it was just hard for me because it's so different from what I would have wanted for my dad.	Dr. L is quietly listening, allowing Dr. R time to reflect and draw his own conclusions.
Dr. L: These situations can be hard to manage.	Again, responds with empathy for the *situation*, explicitly avoiding speaking to the clear (and private!) distress around Dr. R's own belief systems and family.
Dr. L: Would it be okay if we talk about how we might avoid situations like this in the future?	Seeks permission to find a path forward that addresses both party's concerns.
Dr. R: Sure. Do you have any ideas?	
Dr. L: I do, and I'd love to hear yours as well. Do you want me to start?	Shows a willingness to problem solve, making sure that Dr. R knows his ideas will be in the mix.
Dr. R: That would be great.	
Dr. L: Well, my first thought is …	Brainstorming begins.

When Discussing a Conflict Doesn't Go Well

In dealing with conflicts, we would define a successful conversation as one that results in greater understanding on both sides. Note that this does not mean that the conflict will be resolved, because many conflicts won't be over after one good conversation. Real conflicts occur because people have deep commitments, and it takes time to uncover how those commitments can translate into actions that resolve a conflict.

If, after a conversation, you find yourself feeling like you've been in a brawl, first take care of yourself. Take some time to decompress. Ask a colleague you trust to help you think it through. Find a private place to put your own feelings on the table – your frustration, irritation, even sadness. Remember that the things that upset you are probably the things to which you are really committed. We also offer a caveat about the way you mentally review what happened. Instead of rehearsing the reasons you were right, ask yourself if you really understood the other person's thinking. Can you answer the humanizing question about why a well-meaning person is taking this position?

There are some occasions when you should consider apologizing. When the other person feels disrespect from you, an apology is in order. Your original intention is not the point here, and you shouldn't mention it. What you should mention is that you are aware that the other person felt disrespected and that you regret it. When you do apologize, just apologize and make a commitment to try to do better next time. Do not use the occasion to try to make your point again. Do not apologize and end with "but I do think that ... " It's a mark of insincerity and will make the situation worse.

What If the Other Person Doesn't Want to Talk About It?

Sometimes, no matter how safe you attempt to make it and no matter how neutral and even-handed the invitation, the other person just doesn't want to talk about the conflict. Maybe the timing is off or they're still working through their own feelings on the situation. Or, maybe they're just hoping to avoid the conversation altogether. Whatever their reason (and you don't need to know what it is!), our recommendation in that case is that you attend to the emotion of the topic rather than the topic itself. For example, you might say something like, "It seems like this topic has been on both of our minds." It's okay to gently let them know that you hope to discuss it sometime in the future, but don't push. Give them time to regroup, trusting that you've planted seeds just by raising the topic. Then, regroup yourself and take some time to identify your next steps.

What If You Are Feeling Attacked?

Everything we talked about in the "When People Are Rude" section of Chapter 10 applies here as well. Sometimes, though, it feels easier to get pulled into a fight with a colleague than it does with a patient, in part because it can feel more like a personal attack. So, if your colleague is hostile or rude, you may feel justified in responding to them in the same way they treated you. We encourage you to resist that urge. In our experience, that only escalates the argument and makes things worse. Instead, look at their emotion as data (e.g., that anger may represent threat, fear, or anxiety); that will help you decide how to respond next. Remember that the most skilled response you can offer is one that demonstrates empathy for the situation and the people involved.

That does not, however, mean that you need to tolerate abuse or bad behavior. Sometimes, pointing out in a nonjudgmental fashion how threatening or angry the other person seems can help them settle down. For example, it often happens that the object of someone's anger sees the anger much sooner than the person expressing anger. We've all heard the common spousal story in which one spouse loudly declares, "I'm not angry!" in response to their partner asking why they are angry – when what they should probably say instead is, "Oh, I hadn't noticed yet." So, help the other person out – consider gently holding up a mirror so they can see how you perceive their behavior.

For example, you might simply say, "You sound angry" and give them a second to absorb that and settle down. Or, you could say something like, "I really want to sort through this with you, but it is difficult for me to hear you when you lean forward, clench your fists, and raise your voice." Chances are that person has no idea they've become threatening and letting them know will help them make an informed decision about how they wish to proceed professionally.

What if that person can't settle down or you sense that they don't want to? It's always okay to take a break or walk away. No one benefits from you becoming unhinged – especially not you. If you are worried about wasting the other person's time – don't. It will take much more time to clean up a situation made worse by you losing your temper. To extricate yourself politely, you might say something like, "Thanks for sharing your concerns. I'm going to take some time to absorb it, and I'll get back to you when I'm ready to discuss it further," or "Discussing this more now isn't going to be productive. I'm going to take a break, and we'll find another time to finish the discussion." Either of these options allows you to take control of your well-being and both parties time to cool off and regroup.

Finally, these strategies may not be as effective when the conflict is with a colleague with greater institutional power. If one feels that describing the abuse to the other person, or even walking away, puts them at professional risk, doing so may be impossible. Again, in such situations, the only recourse may be to seek out one's supervisor, an ombudsman, or other institutional structure for assistance and support.

When the Relationship Is Still Hard (or the Conflict Seems Unresolvable)

Not all differences of opinion are going to be resolved with alignment, and not all relationships will be as good as you want them to be. That's okay. These are work relationships, and it is entirely possible to be great colleagues without being great friends. You can agree to disagree on many (even most) things and still move forward professionally, particularly as persistent differences of opinion usually reflect divergent core values. Remember, everyone at work is motivated to behave professionally and do the best job they can. Accepting that, even when you don't entirely trust the other person and wish they did certain things differently, can go a long way in having a peaceful, professional working relationship. You don't need to love your boss or colleague (or vice versa) to have a functional and professional working relationship. Work with what you have, recognizing the limits of what is possible.

Sometimes, however, you realize you can't resolve the problem on your own and you need help – even when the conflict is between work equals. Maybe talking to the other person has made things worse – or you find their behavior threatening – and they either can't or won't change it. In such cases, you may need to find a third party to mediate. To minimize contention, framing this as an invitation can reduce the sense of threat ("Could we bring someone who hasn't been involved to help us move forward?"). If that isn't possible and/or the stakes are too high and you feel safety is at risk (e.g., in the case of harassment), you may need to appeal to a higher authority, such as your supervisor, their supervisor, or an institutional resource, like human resources. Obviously, unilaterally going to a higher authority can have substantial relationship consequences, so, for your own sake, such a move should be reserved for only the most dire circumstances.

ACKNOWLEDGING MY PRICKLY SIDE

I was late and feeling overworked, and I had been in a room with a very demanding family. When I walked out of the room, the nurse intercepted me with a look of reproach. We had discussed trying to make sure the family received a consistent message. The nurse started to talk while I was still five feet away, like she didn't think I was going to wait to hear her side of the story. Not hostile – but a little tense. I said, "I do want to acknowledge my role in this. Talking to the family without you was not a good idea. I apologize." To my surprise, she said, "Well, I had not been clear with you either." Acknowledging my contribution quite disarmed her, a bit of repair that got us restarted in a better way.

The Bottom Line

Instead of focusing on being right, work to make things right by reflecting on your own role in the conflict, seeking to understand the other person's side, and working with them to find a shared purpose and mutually acceptable pathway forward.

Maximizing Your Learning

Conflict is tough because afterward we can feel a bit defensive, beat up, or just bad – and the more you value collaboration, the worse you are likely to feel. So be kind to yourself, and remember that you, too, are doing your best. Here are some useful follow-up reflective questions (from Stone, Patton, and Heen) that you can use by yourself, or even better, with a trusted colleague.

- What aspects of your identity or self-image might be threatened? What might you be denying or exaggerating?
- To what extent are you holding yourself to an impossibly high standard?
- How can you regain perspective?
- How can you remember to cut yourself some slack?

Further Reading

Brown, B. *Rising Strong: How the Ability to Reset Transforms the Way We Live, Love, Parent and Lead.* Random House, New York, 2015.

Fisher, R., B. M. Patton, and W. L. Ury, *Getting to Yes: Negotiating Agreement Without Giving In*, 3rd ed. Penguin Books, New York, 2011.

Patterson K., J. Grenny, R. McMillan, and A. Switzler. *Crucial Confrontations: Tools for Resolving Broken Promises, Violated Expectations and Bad Behavior*. McGraw-Hill, New York, 2005.

Stone, D. and Heen, S. *Thanks for the Feedback: The Science and Art of Receiving Feedback Well.* Penguin Group, New York, 2014.

Stone, D., B. Patton, and S. Heen, *Difficult Conversations: How to Discuss What Matters Most*, 2nd ed. Penguin Books, New York, 2010.

12
· · · · · · ·

When You're Really Stuck
Tracking the Talk ... and Adjusting

Why Some Conversations Are Particularly Tough

Up to this point, we have discussed approaches to the most typical serious illness conversations. We've reviewed foundational skills like noticing and responding to emotions as well as strategies for navigating conflict and other difficult situations. In our experience, these skills and roadmaps allow clinicians to confidently manage most conversations they encounter. This chapter focuses on the situations that remain hard, even when you employ all the tools we've already shared. We'll talk about three ways that we think clinicians are commonly stretched as communicators. The first is when the foundational skills might work, but the conversations are difficult because they present rare challenges, have unusually high stakes, or involve heavy emotions. The second is when empathy, the key communication superpower, doesn't work. The third is when our own issues interfere with our ability to be effective. We'll start with two examples of particularly difficult conversations that require mastery of the skills we've already discussed.

Difficult Conversations: Miracles

When a patient or family member says they are hoping for a miracle, it can feel like a conversation stopper. How can you help someone prepare for a bad outcome if they're convinced a higher power will make it go away? In such cases we often hear exasperated clinicians exclaim that the patients or families "just don't get it" and we've observed that attempts to convince them that a miracle won't happen don't go well.

The first thing to appreciate is that, in most cases, patients or families hoping for a miracle do "get it." They know things are bad and that's why a miracle is the only available option. People don't invoke miracles when things are going well. Therefore, your task is not to convince them of the seriousness of the medical situation. Instead, start by attending to the emotion that anyone would be feeling when faced with a situation so desperate that a miracle is necessary (see Chapter 2).

Then, try the following approach:

1. **Explore:** "What would a miracle look like?" We often assume that a miracle means cure, but sometimes we're surprised to find out that a miracle is something that we can help them achieve, like making it to an upcoming wedding or the family arriving in time to say goodbye.
2. **Join:** "We're hoping for that too." Share in the hope for a miracle. It's easy to do because it is true. How wonderful would it be if the illness for which your medical interventions are no longer working suddenly improved?
3. **Expand:** "Are there other things we might hope for?" Even if the hope is for cure, there may be other, more attainable, hopes that patients and families may be thinking about.
4. **Ask:** "Can we talk about what we do if a miracle doesn't happen?" Asking permission to go to a hypothetical space often feels safer and can allow for some exploration and planning.

The following example picks up in the middle of a conversation with the family of an elderly patient in the ICU with pneumonia and multisystem organ failure.

What happened	What we can learn
Mrs. P: You can't give up! We believe in miracles, and I know God is going to step in for Dad.	
Dr. B: We've seen you by his bedside every day. You've done an amazing job supporting him every step of the way.	*Using a support statement to attend to the emotion accompanying this hope for a miracle.*
Mrs. P: Thank you. I know he'd be there for me.	*Feeling heard and calming down.*
Dr. B: You mentioned your hope that Dad will get his miracle. Can I ask what a miracle would look like?	*Exploring.*
Mrs. P: Getting better and being Dad again.	*Hoping for a cure.*
Dr B: We're all hoping and working for that too.	*Sharing in the hope for a miracle.*
Mrs. P: Thank you. Everyone at this hospital has been really great.	
Dr. B: Are there other things we might hope for?	*Seeing if she may be able to expand hopes beyond cure.*
Mrs. P: Well, I want him to be comfortable. When he coughs on the ventilator, it looks so painful!	*Starting to think about other things that are important.*
Dr. B: It must be so hard to see him going through all of this. We'll definitely adjust his medications to keep him as comfortable as possible.	*Attending to her distress and addressing her concerns.*
Mrs. P: Thank you.	
Dr. B: While we're working to get him comfortable and hoping he gets better, I'm wondering if we also might be able to talk about what we do if the miracle doesn't happen. Have you allowed yourself to think about that?	*Sharing hope and asking if she can discuss the hypothetical of what we do if the miracle doesn't happen.*

What happened	What we can learn
Mrs. P: [sighs] I don't like to think about that. We need to be strong and keep praying … but if it doesn't happen … I don't know … I know he wouldn't want to stay like this …	*Starting to engage in a deeper goals conversation.*

It may also be worthwhile to explore the patient's faith and how this plays into the hope for a miracle. Reflecting that "It feels like you have a strong faith" or asking the patient to "Tell me more about what your faith says about miracles" is a way to learn more about the patient's beliefs. In some cases, it might help to talk to the patient's spiritual leader; in others, offering to have the chaplain talk to the patient may provide needed support.

Difficult Conversations: Requests for Hastened Death

A second difficult conversation that stretches even the most seasoned clinicians is when a patient facing a terminal illness asks for help in ending their life. This topic is arising more frequently as medical aid in dying is now legal for almost a third of US citizens, throughout all of Canada, and in multiple other countries around the world. We won't go into the ethical debate about medical aid in dying, as that is beyond the scope of this book. Rather, we'll focus on an approach to the initial request that can be helpful regardless of your own feelings on the topic or whether this is, or is not, a legal option where you practice.

The data suggests that these requests are usually due to a combination of symptoms, debility, loss of sense of self, loss of control, fear of the future, and fear of being a burden. We see these requests as an opportunity to better understand a patient's experience of suffering. While it is certainly important to evaluate decision-making capacity and suicidality, the main conversational task, as with miracles, is to be curious and explore.

We suggest the following approach:

1. *Clarify the question:* Often the initial request for hastened death is phrased in vague terms like, "I want this to be over. Can you help with that?" The first step is to clarify. Try "Tell me exactly what you're asking." In an area as sensitive as this, you want to avoid assumptions. For example, are they asking that we stop treatments that might prolong life, that you be willing to help them end their life in the future, or that you help them do it now?

2. *Express support:* "Thank you for bringing this up. I can see that you've been thinking a lot about this and I appreciate you trusting me to help think this through with you." It is a vulnerable thing to ask a health care provider for help in shortening your life so it's important to begin with reciprocating the patient's trust in you by committing to explore this and find a mutually acceptable solution.

3. *Explore their experience of suffering:* "Tell me more about why you're thinking about this possibility." Explore the multidimensional nature of the suffering behind the request. Remember the concept of total pain with its physical, psychological, social, and spiritual components. In addition, exploring who the patient has spoken with about this and what their friends and family think, may help identify issues that need clarifying. If not already involved, an intradisciplinary specialty palliative care team can help here.

4. *Respond to emotions:* Throughout this conversation, emotions often run high and the NURSE skills discussed in Chapter 2 remain essential.

5. *Negotiate trials of intensifying treatments to alleviate suffering:* If there are reversible elements to their suffering, see if they are willing to let you try addressing them. ("Given that it sounds like the main reason you're wanting this to be over is X, I'm wondering what you'd think about taking some time to see if we can make that better by doing Y.")

6. *Explore whether the patient's concerns might be relieved without aid in dying.* Patients may fear situations that we know are unlikely to happen (e.g., "being a vegetable for months"). All of the authors have seen that explaining more about the dying process, and the available options that do not involve hastened death, often provides significant reassurance and leads patients to no longer feel the need for aid in dying.

7. *Respond directly to the request:* Respond to this honestly within the context of what is legal where you practice and what you are comfortable doing. In many cases, understanding and addressing their suffering and committing to walk this road with them is all that is needed.

When Responding to Emotion Doesn't Change the Conversation

The two difficult conversation types just discussed both required expert use of foundational skills including exploring, asking permission, and, especially, noticing and responding to emotions. The difference between routine conversations and discussions such as these is similar to the difference between dribbling a basketball in your driveway and what a professional player does to blow past an NBA defense. The basic action is the same – dribbling. The pro takes it to a much higher level – faster, stealthier, and more creative. There are some scenarios, however, where the foundational skill of expressing empathy doesn't work, however expertly applied.

Strictly empathic communication fails when the patient actually wants and needs information, not emotional support. As we discussed in Chapter 2, we think of people as having an emotional and a cognitive channel and they are generally only in one channel at a time. One of the most frequent errors we've described is when clinicians hear patients ask for information and assume they are in the cognitive channel, when responding to their emotion first would be far more effective. However, the opposite occurs as well. Sometimes it may appear that the patient is in the emotion channel when they actually want, and need, cognitive information. Consider a patient who hears that there are no further treatments for their pulmonary hypertension and responds with, "There must be something else you can do!" We would generally assume this to be an expression of emotion and respond with something like, "I can't imagine how hard this must be to hear." We would know this form of empathic communication was not working if the patient responded by calmly saying, "Thank you for that, but I've been reading online that there are different treatments depending on the cause of your pulmonary hypertension and I guess I don't understand what is the cause of mine. What is it?" While a response to emotion may come later, in this moment, the clinician must respond to this informational need. Further empathic language would likely only create frustration and a sense of dodging the question.

Another scenario where empathic language may not work is when you need to prioritize containing the emotional chaos. Sometimes, emotions can escalate to the point of aggression or violence. Objects may be thrown, and families may begin yelling at each other or the clinician. This may be especially difficult in the setting of substance abuse, personality disorders, or other mental health conditions that affect behavior. In these situations, if you feel safe, you may start by naming the emotion. However, if things escalate or become unsafe, a containment strategy may be needed. For example, if the patient asking about pulmonary hypertension learns there really are no further treatment options and becomes angry and, despite attempts at expressing empathy, escalates and starts yelling, "Get out! Get out! Get out!", further empathic statements would likely not help. Instead, you may need to prioritize containing the emotional chaos by saying something like, "Let's take a pause. I'm on your side and want to help you with this. How about I come back this afternoon and we can try again to think together about what to do next."

The third common scenario where acknowledging emotion doesn't work is when patients are relying heavily on intellectualization to cope and are focused on finding treatments, often to the exclusion of other coping mechanisms. In these cases, it is often helpful to respect the search first. For example, consider our patient with pulmonary hypertension who says, "There must be something else you can do!" The patient may respond to our attempts at empathy with, "I can't think about stopping right now. I've been talking with a group from Texas. They need to speak with a physician here to know if I qualify for their trial. Can you speak with them?" If the medical situation allows, it may be more productive to respect the search and help them explore this option. This may strengthen your relationship with the patient and help put the serious news in a more understandable context.

These last two examples demonstrate how certain patients may respond to empathic communication quite differently. Some have trouble containing emotions and further empathy causes them to spiral and become much more emotional to the point where it may be unsafe. In these cases, a containment strategy may be needed until the situation is safer. Other patients try very hard to avoid "going there" because they find emotions overwhelming and worry that they will start crying and be unable to stop. They are often highly functioning intellectual problem-solvers who will resist attempts at empathy. You'll recognize this type when you hear things like, "I appreciate your concern, but I need to focus on the problem." Further dwelling in their emotional space will rarely be helpful. In either case, we would recommend bringing in psychosocial expertise and the input of an interdisciplinary team.

When It Feels Close to Home

The other place we see clinicians, including ourselves, stretched as communicators is when the situation triggers our own strong emotions. Sometimes it's in response to a patient's emotion. For example, we often hear that anger is the hardest emotion to manage, and that may be because it's directly threatening to us and, therefore, triggers our own fear. Other times, patients may not act in ways with which we agree, and this spills over, triggering our own frustration. Conversely, some patients do exactly what we want, get worse despite our best efforts, and we may feel some responsibility and all of the emotions that go with seeing someone worsen despite doing everything within our power to stop the disease from progressing. Finally, some clinical situations may remind us of our own past experiences (e.g., a patient dying of cancer who reminds you of a family member who died of the same disease at the same age) and our past emotions resurface.

These emotions are real, and no approach will remove them. Even so, there are some things clinicians can do to remain helpful to their patients even when their own emotions have been triggered. First, try to anticipate how you might feel prior to an interaction. Sometimes knowing the case hits close to home ahead of time can make things more manageable in the moment. It can allow you to bring a team member to help if you get overwhelmed. Knowing it may be hard may also prompt you to practice the interaction ahead of time, so you can be sure you are clear about what you want to achieve and have some words to get started.

You can also bring some tools to help you during the conversation. In real time, pay attention to your own emotions and try to note how they are impacting your thinking. This awareness may allow you to course-correct in the moment. For example, you can use silence to give yourself some time. You can also try addressing the patient's emotions. We've found this often helps calm our own feelings in a tough situation. Another approach is to name our own emotions – although we only do this when we are certain it is in the service of the patient. For example, after giving bad news to a beloved patient one could say "I wish I had better news." One needs to be careful not to redirect the attention to ourselves or make it seem like we're blaming the patient. For example, consider a patient who has been under your care for years and is now dying of multisystem organ failure in the ICU. In meeting with the wife who is tearful, you become very sad because he has worsened despite your treatment, and you are grieving the impending loss of your relationship. To deal with your welling emotion, it may be effective to say, "He did everything we asked of him and it's so hard to see him this way." On the other hand, it may divert attention to say, "He reminds me of my own Dad, and I just can't get over how I failed him when he needed me most!"

If you are feeling overwhelmed, in addition to naming your emotion, it's okay to display what you're feeling, for example, by crying with a patient or family. As in the example above, we try to do this only if it's in line with the tenor of the interaction and, therefore, potentially in the service of the patient or family. If the overwhelming emotions become more about you and may distract from your attempts to help the patient, we suggest excusing yourself and stepping out of the room until you can be the clinician the patient/family needs at that moment. Again, you may need to draw on the help of your team in these most difficult moments.

After an interaction that hits close to home, we have found it essential to debrief with a trusted colleague. Most of us need time and space to unpack such moments and recenter enough to be helpful to the other patients we are seeing. It is also important to track how often such encounters are happening. If it is frequent, it may suggest burnout or other personal issues that may benefit from more direct interventions like counseling.

BOX: SHARING TEARS

Recently, I was a palliative care consultant for a patient with cancer who had been in the hospital for weeks with numerous complications and was now actively dying. I joined a family meeting with the primary team where we discussed comfort-focused care. The family began to cry and the resident, who had cared for the patient for the whole month, cried with them. They embraced and everyone calmed and left the room with what felt like a palpable sense of being heard, understood, and cared for. Afterwards, the resident apologized profusely for crying, yet, in my subsequent meetings with the family, they couldn't speak highly enough of the care she had provided for the patient. It was an important reminder of how, despite a medical culture that often discourages emotional connections, sharing tears is almost always appreciated and seen as evidence of how much you value the person and how invested you are in their care.

The Bottom Line

In hard conversations, start by responding to emotion but track the patient's and your own responses and alter your approach as needed.

Maximizing Your Learning

Seek out a course to try rare/challenging scenarios in a safe learning environment. We generally learn new and challenging skills best by practicing them in a low-stakes setting. Opportunities to receive observation and feedback, particularly when working with patient actors, can be enormously helpful. If such a course is not available, you can always ask a colleague to role-play with you a potentially challenging encounter.

Further Reading

Back, A. L. and R. M. Arnold, "Isn't there anything more you can do?": When empathic statements work, and when they don't. *J Palliat Med*, 2013, **16**(11): 1429–32.

Cooper, R. S., A. Ferguson, J. N. Bodurtha, and T. J. Smith, AMEN in challenging conversations: Bridging the gaps between faith, hope, and medicine. *J Oncol Pract* 2014, **10**(4): e191–5.

Posluszny, D. and R. M. Arnold, Managing one's emotions as a clinician. *J Palliat Med*, 2009, **12**(10): 955–6.

Quill, T. E., A. L. Back, and S. D. Block, Responding to patients requesting physician-assisted death: Physician involvement at the very end of life. *JAMA*, 2016, **315**(3): 245–6.

Widera, E. W., K. E. Rosenfeld, E. K. Fromme, D. P. Sulmasy, and R. M. Arnold, Approaching patients and family members who hope for a miracle. *J Pain Symptom Manage*, 2011, **42**(1): 119–25.

13
· · · · · · ·

Talking about Dying
"Do Not Resuscitate" Orders and Goodbyes

How You Talk about Dying Makes a Difference

Talking about dying can be one of the most frustrating and stressful communication tasks or, paradoxically, one of the most satisfying. The reasons for frustration are formidable: patients are "not ready," "in denial," or "unrealistic." The reasons for deep satisfaction are equally impressive, in a different way. Clinicians describe the experience of talking to dying patients as a "privilege," "life-changing," or "amazing." What accounts for the divergence? Certainly, patients vary considerably in their willingness and capacity to talk about their own impending death. In addition, different cultures have different ways of talking about death. Yet, in our experience, the most powerful variable surrounding discussions of dying is the clinician rather than the patient. If you practice the roadmaps in this chapter, you could change your experience of talking about dying from chronically frustrating and stressful to commonly rewarding and even transformative.

Why Is Talking about Dying So Tricky?

The communication tasks in this chapter might be the most difficult, but for completely different reasons. While most clinicians have lots of experience talking with patients about resuscitation preferences (commonly called "talking about cardiopulmonary resuscitation [CPR]" or "do not resuscitate [DNR] orders"), many have never seen the roadmap we recommend. Furthermore, when it comes to discussing end of life concerns and saying goodbye to patients, many clinicians have minimal training. These two moments – talking about resuscitation preferences and clinicians preparing patients for the end and saying goodbye – represent important touchstones in a patient–clinician relationship.

Working in the Shadow of Death

In our VitalTalk workshops, one of the most powerful insights we observe is that clinicians hesitate to bring up dying because they know it will raise strong emotions, from the patient, the family, and themselves, and they're not sure what to do with these. Their hesitation to talk about death then serves as an unintended model for how the patient and family should deal with dying – by avoiding it. The kind of professional development that is required to overcome this hesitancy goes beyond learning a communication skill. Clinicians who harbor these worries need to develop more capacity to be in the presence of their own strong emotions and those of their patients. (You can learn it, although most medical training doesn't address it.) Unfortunately, clinicians don't always recognize that they are avoiding the emotion. Their learned avoidance happens so fast that they are unaware of it. What they do notice is that their interactions with patients and families get stuck again and again. We will have more to say about how to develop this capacity, a personal sort of emotional intelligence, in the next chapter. But here we want to say that developing your capacity to hold space for emotion is a long-term project, and in the short term, it can help to have another person who can help you deal with the emotion. This may be another member of your team, and frequently someone from a different discipline.

> **The Pitfall:** Hesitating to bring up death because the emotion will be too much.
>
> **The Solution:** Find a colleague to sit with you in the visit, and expand your own capacity to deal with strong emotion.

Bucking a "Death-Denying" Culture?

Many patients and families have little first-hand experience with the process of dying. They've seen CPR work on television (where the resuscitated patient lives for another episode more than two-thirds of the time); they've seen the ads from your medical center promising miracles with the newest technology; they know about Lance Armstrong's battle with cancer that preceded his winning the Tour de France seven times (even if he had a little help from doping!); and they've heard about someone who has woken up from a coma after years of being unresponsive. Your patients live in a culture that Kathleen Foley called "death-denying." For you, performing CPR on a dying patient may feel like an assault and violate your notion of a "good death." Yet, when you talk to patients about forgoing resuscitation for a better death, you look like the outlier, or worse, someone who has given up on them or doesn't value them enough to try everything possible.

We have great sympathy for clinicians who have been fired by patients because they talked too much about dying, because we've been there. Because of our clinical experience, we are often thinking several steps ahead of the patient and family. Talking about dying requires that the patient and family be willing and able to think about the medical treatment not working. Elisabeth Kubler-Ross talked about the "stages" of adjusting to death – denial, bargaining, anger, grief, and acceptance – and while patients do not necessarily follow this exact sequence, this work reminds us that acknowledgment is a process. And if they have not accepted the possibility of death, then it is very unlikely that they will consider not performing a "life-saving" treatment like CPR.

The mark of an accomplished communicator in this context is to create a conversation (or series of conversations) in which the patient and family absorb the information and gradually create their own vision of the future. You need to guide patients and families to a deeper realization of the medical situation at a speed that they can cognitively and emotionally tolerate.

Our own biases about discussing death, likely formed from challenging experiences in our past, also interfere with our ability to comfortably enter this space. It may be helpful to pause and remember that each situation is different, granting each person the respect of acknowledging their own unique story. With increasing public conversations about the topic, your patient may also surprise you by not being so "death denying" after all. Multiple organizations have worked to normalize discussions about death in the community, including Death Over Dinner and Death Cafe. Articles about end-of-life issues are common in the media, and books such as *Being Mortal* by Atul Gawande have become part of our popular culture. Of course, talking about death intellectually is different than facing it oneself. Yet these cultural influences have likely made it easier for many patients to broach the topic with a clinician. Given the variability of each person's experience, consider approaching the conversation with a sense of curiosity rather than bracing for disaster. Clinicians may be setting themselves up for unnecessary stress if they don't pay attention to their internal monologue and practice patterns.

Don't Use DNR Orders to Introduce Dying

Most patients and families need time to understand and adapt to the changing reality of approaching death. Backing into the conversation about dying from a DNR discussion is not only awkward, but it does not offer the patient the opportunity to first come to terms with their own mortality. It may seem easier to talk about dying only when a patient's body is failing or a team member prompts you to write a DNR order. But the downside of procrastination is that too much work is left to be done in too short a period of time. For the patient and family this sudden transition to understanding that they are dying can feel rapid and overwhelming. In this scenario, patients have viewed their medical team as reassuring cheerleaders, only to suddenly see them turn, as one family member put it, "completely negative."

This is also the reason to start first, perhaps much earlier in the serious illness, with a conversation about goals of care, and to allow the DNR discussion to evolve naturally from that. The pitfall clinicians fall into is to talk about restarting a disembodied organ without anchoring the discussion in the patient's big picture or their values. "Do you want us to do restart your heart if it stops?" "Give pressors?" "Intubate?" This entire strategy may be an unintended consequence of ethical guidelines that stress the importance of patient autonomy and choice in talking about resuscitation at the end of life. Unfortunately, in practice, many clinicians have reduced this to "going in to get the DNR order."

Unfortunately, many patients feel terribly vulnerable near death, have a strong sense of their dependence on medical technology (it's kept them alive thus far), and fear being abandoned by their health care providers. Therefore, our cognitive roadmap for DNR orders is really the roadmap for late-stage goals of care discussions, and includes making a recommendation about what should (and should not) be done based on what informed patients have said is important to them. Once you've articulated what you will do to care for the patient, only then do you make a recommendation about CPR, linking your recommendation to the patient's values.

The Pitfall: Asking separately about every component of resuscitation.

The Solution: Guide the patient by developing the big picture, talking about the care plan, and making a recommendation about CPR as one element of the larger care plan.

Roadmap for Discussing Resuscitation Preferences (DNR Discussions)

Using the REMAP framework (introduced in Chapter 8 for late-stage goals of care), DNR can be part of a larger conversation in which we first elicit the patient's understanding and goals and then make a recommendation about care that includes consideration of CPR. To some, this approach to a DNR order may seem indirect. But this conversation is not about filling out a form or offering all possible interventions in a value-neutral way; you need to align your recommendations with the patient's values. This approach is far more patient-centered than asking someone, out of context, whether they "want" to be resuscitated.

1. *Elicit the patient's understanding of their illness.* This is the recurring theme of leading conversations with Ask-Tell-Ask. Even if you have a long-standing relationship and an assumed shared understanding, it may be helpful to ascertain how they think things are going with their illness now.
2. *Discuss the "big picture" of what's happening medically.* By "big picture," we mean the "headline" – a global view of the situation. You may need to provide a reframe that the medical condition has progressed.
3. *Respond to emotion.* This skill can never be omitted in any conversation that involves serious news.
4. *Ask about patient values in context.* A typical question might be, "Given your medical situation, what is most important to you?" Sometimes people focus immediately on "I want to live," especially if they have had repetitive code status conversations. Of course, they want to live! The better question might be, "Whenever the time comes that you are at the end of your life, what would be important?" or, "If time is short, how do you want to spend it?"
5. *Make a recommendation about DNR as part of the care plan.* Aligning with the patient's stated priorities, discuss things you would do before discussing interventions you would stop or not initiate. Make a recommendation about DNR as the last part of the care plan. *Explicitly* link your recommendations to the patient's values and perceptions elicited earlier and ask what they think. It is not necessary to ask for permission for each intervention and it is generally preferred to describe resuscitation as a package. If you must

cover specific interventions (doing so is a requirement in New York State, for example), you can simply describe what your recommendation covers in enough detail to fill out the required form.

6. *Be prepared, again, to respond to emotion.*

7. *Tell the patient that you will document the conversation and write an order.* Explain that the order can be changed at any time. Remind the patient and family that medical care will continue, as patients are worried about being abandoned. If your hospital uses DNR wristbands or signs, it may be good to let the patient know about this to avoid an unwelcome surprise. This may also be the time to complete or update a POLST form (or equivalent). Some patients are tired or even traumatized by repetitive code status conversations, especially those detached from any discussion of their values. Completing a POLST form allows the patient to point to it and tell the next health-care provider (or 10) that their wishes are the same, and it gives the patient a place to start if their situation or goals have changed.

Example Discussion

Here's part of a conversation between a patient with advanced cancer who has been receiving chemotherapy and has been hospitalized for pneumonia – we're picking up the conversation midstream, after the physician has already assessed the patient's understanding.

WHAT HAPPENED	WHAT WE CAN LEARN
Dr. Y: I'm glad to see that your pneumonia seems to be stabilizing. Could we change topics now and talk for a few minutes about the overall care plan? I'd like to make some recommendations and get your feedback.	*Using signposting to denote a change of topics. Framing recommendations as asking a patient for feedback.*
Ms. C: Okay.	

WHAT HAPPENED	WHAT WE CAN LEARN
Dr. Y: I'm hoping that we've turned the corner on this pneumonia and that you'll continue to improve. That's the best-case scenario, and I will do everything possible to make that happen.	*Giving the big picture of the medical situation.*
Ms. C: Thank you, that is what I am hoping for too.	
Dr. Y: I would also like to be prepared for the possibility that things do not go the way we hoped. I know this can be tough to talk about.	*Giving rationale for talking about dying that involves the doctor (not only the patient) – I want to be prepared – and acknowledging difficulty. Note that "Hope for the best, prepare for the worst" is implicit in this comment.*
Ms. C: I *would* like to be prepared. …	
Dr. Y: What are the things that come to your mind when you say you want to be prepared?	*Eliciting patient concerns.*
Ms. C: Well, I want my husband to be able to accept this; he is having a hard time.	
Dr. Y: That's important. Is there anything else?	
Ms. C: Umm, I would like to talk to my daughter and son but I'm not sure what to say.	
Dr. Y: Also very important. How much have you been thinking about dying?	*Asking explicitly about dying as he has only alluded to this previously.*
Ms. C: A bit. Of course, I know it will happen to all of us.	
Dr. Y: That's true. When you think about your death, what would you like it to be like?	*Asking for patient wishes.*

WHAT HAPPENED	WHAT WE CAN LEARN
Ms. C: I would like it to be peaceful, and comfortable. I'd like to be at home.	
Dr. Y: Those are very helpful things for me to know because I can do a much better job for you. Based on what you have told me, could I make some recommendations now?	*Reinforcing the rationale to talk with the patient about dying. Asking permission to make recommendations.*
Ms. C: Yes.	
Dr. Y: We just talked about the best-case scenario for what's happening. I'd like to talk about the worst-case scenario, too. If this pneumonia got worse, we would normally consider moving you to the intensive care unit and even putting you on a breathing machine. But the risk of doing that is that you could end up dying in the ICU. And given all that's going on with your health, it would almost certainly not be successful. If you would like to be at home, and have as peaceful a death as possible, I would recommend that if things got worse that we should try to set up you home with the right kind of care, so that you could spend as much time at there as possible. Does that make sense to you?	*Making a recommendation about the worst-case scenario.*
Ms. C: Yes it does.	
Dr. Y: I would also recommend that we focus on your comfort at the time of death, and not do CPR. I don't think CPR would help you have a peaceful death at home. What do you think about that?	
Ms. C: I thought CPR could bring me back.	

WHAT HAPPENED	WHAT WE CAN LEARN
Dr. Y: Well, it does look like that on TV. But in reality, if the cancer is the problem, CPR doesn't change the cancer.	
Ms. C: I see what you mean.	

This is only a brief excerpt from this conversation, and we would expect that this doctor and patient might continue to talk more and might circle around again through the issues. However, we think that keeping the focus on the big picture, and using an implicit "Hope for the best, prepare for the worst" philosophy are useful underlying principles for these discussions.

When the End of Life Is Getting Closer

As patients approach the end of life, they and their caregivers may have questions that go unasked. When clinicians create the space to talk and hear these concerns, we may be able to address uncertainty and suffering that otherwise would have remained hidden.

One of the easiest things we can do to start this conversation is to just ask, "Tell me what worries you. What's keeping you up at night?" Normalizing the concerns around illness and dying can enable positive coping and may help your patient deal with any stigma they associate with their chronic illness.

Many people report that they worry about dying but don't bring it up or, when they do, do so indirectly. If it seems like everyone is talking around the issue of death, it may be helpful to test the waters by saying, "Many people wonder if it's okay to talk about dying. How much are you thinking about it?" This opens the door for patients to ask questions or express worries in a nonjudgmental way.

This is particularly important for families whose loved ones are dying. They may have never seen anyone die and be unsure what to even ask. Saying, "Would it be helpful for me to describe what you may see over the next few days to weeks?" might allow them to voice their curiosity. Remember to check with all family members because while some might want to hear about the process, others may want to step out.

Other patients feel that they may be blamed for behaviors that may have contributed to their illness, such as alcohol, drug, or tobacco use. This stigma may deter them from seeking support and may worsen their quality of life. Being aware of the potential of a history of mistreatment due to stigma, or a patient's own feelings of guilt or shame, will help you more sensitively address their concerns and questions, and may help them feel listened to without judgment. A useful question in this setting might be, "Are there any aspects of this you find hard to talk about?"

Patients with challenging social histories may also have been victims of various types of trauma, and posttraumatic symptoms and behaviors may become particularly salient toward the end of life. These may include intense feelings of guilt or regret, or worsened flashbacks and nightmares. Care of such patients should allow them to maintain as much control as possible. Listen carefully for clues that the patient may be thinking about their death and ask permission to gently explore with a statement such as, "I wonder if you would want to share what worries you about dying." How to respond fully to such clinical challenges is beyond the scope of this book, but it's useful to be sensitive to this possibility, and to consult someone with expertise in trauma-informed care.

As they get closer to death, many people fear unrelieved symptoms or loss of control. Others fear death itself. Still others are afraid of what will happen after they die, either to their loved ones or to their soul. Their answer will help you focus your response to their actual concerns and will help you know when to bring in additional team members, such as a spiritual care provider.

Creating opportunities to have conversations about spiritual and existential issues, meaning and purpose, and life closure also becomes more urgent. If you have been following this patient over time, you may have already had such discussions. But, if not, opening up a dialogue may allow you to address quiet suffering or create space for your patient to experience personal growth despite their physical decline. "Are you at peace?" is a simple question that can open the door to talking about emotional, spiritual, or existential distress.

Spiritual assessment is an important element of any medical history and becomes even more relevant at end of life. Several tools, such as the FICA (Faith, belief, meaning; Importance and influence; Community; Address, action in care) and HOPE (Sources of Hope; Organized religion; Personal spirituality and practice; Effects on medical care and End of life) have been developed to assist with spiritual assessment and can be useful here. In patients nearing death, you may wish to ask about specific practices or rituals so the medical team is prepared to support the spiritual needs of the patient and family. Finally, inquiring about preferences for place of death not only helps for planning, but may be even more important if some end-of-life practices are difficult or impossible in a health care facility (e.g., not disturbing the body for a certain period of time).

One fairly frequent source of distress arises after a decision has been made to focus on comfort, and the patient takes longer than expected to die. In our experience, this is most common after decisions to stop dialysis or to withhold nutrition and hydration in a severely incapacitated patient. We have personally seen such patients live up to three weeks and this time can be either a blessing or a curse for families. Some families use it as a time to come together, recall memories and accomplishments, express gratitude, and make meaning of their loved one's life and loss. Others are distressed at waiting for the inevitable and seem to find minimal meaning in the time between the decision to stop disease-directed therapy and the patient's death. By listening, providing education, and normalizing the dying process, clinicians create emotional safety and knowledge about what to expect.

Additionally, normalizing the variability in the dying process may help patients and families who begin to doubt their decision-making if the patient outlives the anticipated prognosis. Clinicians can also support patients and families who are struggling by assisting them in life review and in how to say goodbye. For example, you may suggest that they tell stories about the patient, decorate the room with memories, or play the patient's favorite music. You could also say, "Some families find it helpful to say things to the patient like, 'I love you,' 'I forgive you,' 'Please forgive me,' and 'Thank you.'" Finally, you should make clear that we cannot predict the time of death and prepare families for the possibility that this last phase could be much longer than expected. While it may not ease the pain, it will at least eliminate the surprise.

Saying Goodbye to Patients Whom You Do Not Expect to See Again

Think about the patient you saw for one last time in the hospital before discharging him to hospice. Did you say goodbye or acknowledge that this was likely the last time you would see him? Many clinicians avoid these goodbyes. Unfortunately, not acknowledging this moment can leave patients and families feeling abandoned.

Clinicians give a variety of reasons for avoiding goodbyes. We may be concerned about the impact on patients or families: acknowledging we will not see a patient again makes it clear that she is dying and will make her sad. We may worry that patients will feel abandoned or that we are giving up. Prognostic uncertainty also plays a role. We cannot be sure that the patient will not be readmitted next week, which could result in an awkward encounter. Finally, it's hard to say goodbye, and many clinicians worry that they will get emotional and that showing our own emotions may be interpreted as being unprofessional. These personal reactions reflect embedded cultural values about dealing with loss and the role of medicine. Medicine emphasizes cure, and neither clinicians nor their patients like to be reminded that medicine is frequently less than curative. For all these reasons, we often discharge patients without ever acknowledging the sadness and loss running just beneath the small talk.

By ignoring the end of the relationship, clinicians miss an important opportunity. Saying goodbye can have a powerful positive effect. By saying goodbye, we both acknowledge the end of the relationship and at the same time underscore its importance, leaving the patient with a sense of feeling valued and cared for rather than abandoned. Saying goodbye also gives the patient an opportunity to say thank you and to look back over the course of a relationship. For clinicians – especially those in training – a goodbye can be an opportunity to tell patients how they have contributed to that professional's learning and how it will help other patients in the future.

How might one go about saying goodbye? The following roadmap provides a guide:

1. *Choose an appropriate time and place.* A setting that affords some privacy will make it easier to be personal. The end of the visit may seem like a natural time to say goodbye, but if you've had a long, rich relationship with a patient, plan enough time so that there is time for a correspondingly rich and meaningful goodbye.

2. *Acknowledge the end of your routine contact.* This names that you will not be making future appointments and sets the stage for a conversation about closure. ("This may be the last time we get to see each other, so I wanted to say goodbye.")

3. *Invite the patient to respond and use that response as a piece of data about the patient's state of mind.* Saying "Would that be okay?" or "How would you feel about that?" enables patients to have a bit of control over the conversation, and allows them to gather their thoughts. It also enables clinicians to assess patients' willingness to talk about the topic and their emotional frame of mind.

4. *Frame the goodbye as an appreciation.* We think clinicians can use a goodbye opportunity most powerfully by citing something that you truly appreciate about that patient, something that gives the person a sense that you knew them as more than a diagnosis. Some examples: "I just wanted to say how

much I've enjoyed you and how much I've appreciated your flexibility (or cooperation, good spirits, courage, honesty, directness, collaboration) and your good humor (or your insights, thoughtfulness, love for your family)." If it seems appropriate, the clinician can acknowledge the loss of the relationship: "I'll miss seeing you in clinic and hearing about your grandchildren and your husband."

5. *Give space for the patient to reciprocate*, and respond empathically to the patient's emotion. Acknowledging loss and death can make even well-adjusted, high-functioning patients (and clinicians) anxious, and this might be something to acknowledge: "I realize this might seem awkward, but I wanted to make sure that you knew how I felt, rather than risk not having the chance to tell you."

   In our experience, patients often talk about how much they appreciate the clinician's time, effort, and concern. These positive statements may be particularly hard when we may be feeling guilty that our medicines could not do more for the patient. If patients do express appreciation, it is important to receive their comments without minimizing them. Say "Thank you" rather than "It was nothing." The patient is giving you a gift, and it is important that you receive and appreciate it. Not doing so may leave that person feeling unheard or feeling the relationship was unappreciated.

6. *Articulate an ongoing commitment to the patient's care*, to make it clear the patient is not being abandoned. Consider saying something like, "Of course you know I remain available to you and that you can still call me. Your hospice nurse will keep me informed about what is happening. I will be here if you need me, and I'll be thinking about you."

7. *Later, reflect on your work with this particular patient*. Many clinicians received the hidden curriculum that death ought not be discussed much, that clinicians cope by being silent and strong, and that avoiding talk about death is part of self-preservation. We observe that many clinicians have involuntary reflexive responses that may not serve their professional work and personal growth. Developing a conscious awareness of these responses to a patient's death is an important tool. It may be worth asking oneself: "What do I want to take away from taking care of this person?" Because the meaning clinicians assign to their work shapes their professional identities, reflecting on that meaning can help them grow as healers.

Example Conversation

Again, we pick up a conversation midway.

WHAT HAPPENED	WHAT WE CAN LEARN
Tanya, NP: So I think we've covered everything for today. I will ask the hospice to call you tomorrow, and if you don't hear from them, please call us.	*Finishing the medical business before starting a goodbye.*
Mr. G: Okay.	
Tanya, NP: There is one more thing.	
Mr. G: What's that?	
Tanya, NP: I will make an appointment for you to come back in two to three weeks, to see how you are doing. If it is too much work to come in, you can just call us. So, if I don't see you in person again, I want to make sure you know that I've enjoyed working with you. I admire your spirit. Thank you.	*Acknowledging that future contact is uncertain but possible. Framing goodbye as an appreciation.*
Mr. G: Well … thank you too. I don't think I would have had this much time without you. And I have felt well cared for.	*Giving space for the patient to reciprocate.*
Tanya, NP: You are welcome. That means a lot to me. Now, remember, I will still be available if you need me; I'm just a phone call away.	*Responding to the patient's appreciation. Articulating an ongoing commitment to the patient's care.*
Mr. G: I am thankful for that.	
Tanya, NP: You take care, now.	

Not every relationship with a patient who is near death affords an opportunity for saying goodbye. Clinicians need to have established a level of mutual understanding with their patients about the severity of the illness and have some confidence in their ability to deal with sadness, loss, and grief. Acknowledging the end and saying goodbye is best suited for patients who would welcome a moment of feeling connected to their clinician. These conversations may not always be smooth or predictable, but they can nonetheless be deeply meaningful.

At times, a strong bond is formed between clinicians and the patient's caregiver, and saying goodbye and expressing gratitude to your patient's family member is similar to saying goodbye to a patient. Sometimes the goodbye to a patient's significant other happens on the phone after the patient dies. In addition to expressing gratitude for the relationship, praising the family for their caregiving efforts, and making sure they know how to access bereavement counseling services, are important elements to consider. Writing condolence letters and even attending funerals are practices that we support and can also bring benefit for both families and clinicians. However, as they are not direct face-to-face communication, we do not cover them in this book.

Finally, after a patient's death, notifying a colleague who shared in their care is important so your colleague can also reach out to the family with their condolences. Doing so also allows you to express gratitude to your colleague for their care of the patient and for their collaboration with you. It may also serve as a check-in, to create space for shared reflection. Your colleague may be self-critical or may be pleased with the care they provided. They may also be grieving. Sharing a short time of reflection about a patient who has died allows clinicians to give and receive their own emotional support and gratitude.

The Bottom Line

Conducting goals-based discussions about resuscitation prefer-ences is a critical skill when approaching the end of a serious illness. Saying goodbye is an advanced skill for talking to patients, and can be tremendously rewarding.

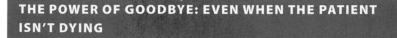

THE POWER OF GOODBYE: EVEN WHEN THE PATIENT ISN'T DYING

Earlier in my career, I decided to focus my clinical practice on palliative care, which meant closing my HIV practice. I was saying goodbye to a woman with HIV for whom I had cared for over 12 years. When we first met, she was addicted to street drugs and weighed 95 pounds. I told her how much she had taught me about second chances and turning one's life around. Then, she surprised me by telling me how much my support meant to her. When faced with something difficult, she would imagine me and what I would say – a way of using my support even when I wasn't there. I had no idea that I had played such a big role in her recovery. The memory of her words has gotten me through some difficult conversations, when I wonder how much of an impact I really have.

Maximizing Your Learning

1. For discussing DNR skills, this roadmap involves a paradigm shift in how to conduct the conversation for clinicians who have only seen the other method. If you have not seen this approach used before, it may be worth watching someone else model this roadmap. When you do, take notes. Make two columns on your piece of paper, and on the left put "What they said," and on the right, put "What I noticed" (about facial expressions, where they looked, what the patient's emotions felt like, what my emotions felt like). Then identify one thing you want to try.

2. To say goodbye, one must anticipate when this might come up and be ready for the conversation. Commit to looking over your clinic or rounding schedule with this in mind and plan with one or two patients to offer an appreciation – even if it's not in the context of saying goodbye. You may find the act of appreciating a patient or family powerful in its own right, and it will serve as practice for saying goodbye.

Further Reading

Back, A. L. R. M. Arnold, J. A. Tulsky, W. F. Baile, and K. A. Fryer-Edwards, On saying goodbye: Acknowledging the end of the patient–physician relationship with patients who are near death. *Ann Intern Med*, 2005, **142**(8): 682–5.

Block, S. D., Perspectives on care at the close of life: Psychological considerations, growth, and transcendence at the end of life: The art of the possible. *JAMA*, 2001, **285**(22): 2898–905.

Byock, I., *The Four Things That Matter Most*. New York, Simon and Schuster, 2014.

Casarett, D. J. and T. E. Quill, "I'm not ready for hospice": Strategies for timely and effective hospice discussions. *Ann Intern Med*, 2007, **146**(6): 443–9.

Chapple, A., S. Ziebland, and A. McPherson, Stigma shame and blame experienced by patients with lung cancer: A qualitative study. *BMJ*, 2004, **328**(7454): 1470.

Gawande, Atul, *Being Mortal: Medicine and What Matters in the End*. New York, Metropolitan Books, 2014.

Hebert R. S., R. Schultz, V. Copeland, and R. M. Arnold, What questions do family caregivers want to discuss with health care providers in order to prepare for the death of a loved one? An ethnographic study of caregivers of patients at end of life. *J Palliat Med*, 2008, **11**(3): 476–83.

Maciejewski, P. K., B. Zhang, S. D. Block, and H. G. Prigerson, An empirical examination of the stage theory of grief. *JAMA*, 2007, **297**(7): 716–23.

Martinez, M., M. Arantzamendi, and A. Belar, "Dignity therapy," a promising intervention in palliative care: A comprehensive systematic literature review. *Palliat Med*, 2017, **31**(6): 492–509.

Prigerson, H. G. and S. C. Jacobs, Perspectives on care at the close of life. Caring for bereaved patients: "All the doctors just suddenly go." *JAMA*, 2001, **286**(11): 1369–76.

Quill, T. E. and C. K. Cassel, Nonabandonment: A central obligation for physicians. *Ann Intern Med*, 1995, **122**(5): 368–74.

Shanafelt, T., A. Adjei, and F. L. Meyskens, When your favorite patient relapses: Physician grief and well-being in the practice of oncology. *J Clin Oncol*, 2003, **21**(13): 2616–19.

Steinhauser, K. E., E. Clipp, and M. McNeilly, In search of a good death: Observations of patients, families, and providers. *Ann Intern Med*, 2000, **132**(10): 825–32.

Steinhauser, K. E., C. I. Voils, and E. C. Clipp, "Are you at peace?" One item to probe spiritual concerns at end of life. *Arch Intern Med*, 2006, **166**(1): 101–05.

von Gunten, C. F., Fast Facts and Concepts #149: Teaching the family what to expect when the patient is dying. www.mypcnow.org/fast-fact/teaching-the-family-what-to-expect-when-the-patient-is-dying/, 2015.

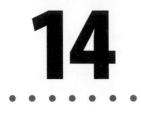

14

Cultivating Your Skills
Bring Your Full Self to the Patient

If you've read this far, you are seriously motivated to do better. And you also know that simply reading about communication is not enough. Improving in a domain as complex as human interaction requires an ongoing commitment and a training process to getting better. In this chapter, we want to share some tools that we hope will help you become a lifelong learner and achieve mastery. We'd love to be at your side coaching you but, given that we can't quite pull that off, hopefully these tips will help you do it on your own and take you to the next level.

We will first focus on how you can become proficient at the skills and roadmaps we've presented throughout this book. We hope you can find practical ways to build this ongoing self-improvement practice into your clinical work. We will then focus on the personal qualities, or capacities, that you bring to this work, and that help you bring your fullest authentic self to clinical encounters. We will explore how you can build on your existing strengths and gain new ones, and thereby create a practice that fosters resiliency.

Mastering Skills and Cognitive Roadmaps

The process of improving any skill, whether it's a sport, an art, or even yo-yo tricks, requires three steps. One needs to observe what "good" looks like, practice the new approach, and receive feedback on how they did. James remembers spending hours in his room as an 11-year-old learning to make his yo-yo "spin around the world," "walk the dog," or "rock the baby." He started by studying the illustrated pages of the *Giant Book of Duncan Yo-Yo Tricks* and then practiced with the yo-yo while repeatedly glancing back at the drawings. Feedback was straightforward – the trick either worked or didn't – although sometimes he asked his big brother to help figure out what he was doing wrong. The key moment arrived when he showed off the new skills to his school friends and enjoyed the accolades that followed. He even started teaching others these tricks, which only made him better himself. Hand James a yo-yo today and he'll show you that enough time spent learning a skill, even 50 years ago, creates lasting muscle memory.

In Chapter 1, we described several habits that build on these principles of observation, practice, and feedback that can support the ongoing learning of communication skills (see "Learning Habits That Set You Up for Success"). At the end of every subsequent chapter, we included brief exercises that would help with maximizing your learning. By now, you should be familiar with picking just one skill at a time to learn, the value of practice, and the importance of feedback. Here, we would like to dive a little deeper into two techniques that can help achieve these results.

LEARNING HABITS THAT SET YOU UP FOR SUCCESS

- ▶ Record yourself
- ▶ Refine your observational skills
- ▶ Practice one new skill at a time

LEARNING HABITS THAT SET YOU UP FOR SUCCESS (CONT.)

▶ Debrief yourself

▶ Ask for feedback

▶ Be patient

▶ Pay attention to praise

The first technique takes advantage of all those moments when we walk into a patient room with another clinician. Before you walk into the room, tell your colleague that you're working on your communication skills and will be looking for feedback. Let them know exactly what you're working on and ask them to observe how you do (or do not) display that skill. You can even encourage your colleague to take notes to get down the exact words you use. For example, perhaps you want to practice making more direct empathic statements, or make sure you ask for a patient's understanding before delivering medical information. Then, after you've left the room, take three minutes to debrief. You should start by sharing how you thought things went and whether you were able to effectively employ the identified skill. Ask your colleague to comment by telling you what they thought you did well (ideally with a description of the exact words) and the impact it had on the encounter. Then ask them to suggest one thing you could do differently next time. If there was a particular point you were curious about, ask them to focus their attention there. The more specific they can be and the more you can discuss exact words to use next time, the more useful these debriefs will feel. Finish off by sharing one thing you took away from the encounter that you'll try to use the next time you're in a similar situation.

The second strategy is more difficult and requires a bit of practice. Learn to observe yourself in real time. Pay attention to what you're doing while you're doing it, watch the reaction of the patient or family, and respond with course corrections, if necessary. We like to think about this as if there is a "mini-me" looking down on the encounter from a corner of the room and giving you feedback as you move along. This may sound like a crazy proposition, but we can attest that it's doable. It requires slowing down a bit, taking pauses when necessary, and a practiced sense of self-awareness. Early on, you may not be able to change what you're doing in the moment (you have to think quickly!), but this practice will heighten your ability to reflect. After the encounter, spend a few minutes replaying it in your head, celebrating a success, and thinking about what you can try next time. By doing so, the next time you find yourself in a similar moment, hopefully you'll be ready with the right words.

Notice Where You Get Stuck and What You Avoid

Are there certain kinds of patients or situations that seem to always be challenging? Do you ever feel like you're in a loop of difficult communication that you don't know how to break? If this happens enough, the natural reaction is to avoid these situations. When you start noticing that similar situations cause problems, think about the common features that are not working and what you might be able to do differently.

When we teach, one of the most common stuck points we observe is when clinicians know what to say but have trouble actually speaking the words. The issue is not the lack of skill, but internal capacities which limit our ability to say the words. For example, one of us was consulting on a 65-year-old man, dying of multisystem organ failure in the ICU. Before the family conference, the ICU attending told the team that the "right thing to do" was to focus on comfort because the patient was "dying." But during the conference, the same attending told the patient's daughter and grandchildren that he was "very sick," that his ICU stay "might not go well," that the ICU team was "very worried" – but did not say he was dying. Consequently, the family asked the team to keep "trying everything." After the meeting, we debriefed the attending who said, in a soft voice, "It's just so sad. They wanted so badly for him to get better." This kind of sadness experienced by a clinician – that prevented this physician from articulating a difficult truth – is something we've experienced ourselves. Our own emotions turn up like popup ads on websites, blocking the real message. Focusing on words and maps alone may fall short in these moments. We must cultivate a different sort of expertise.

Building Capacities

In Chapter 1, we described capacities as the character elements that clinicians bring to each encounter. They allow us to both be our full authentic selves with our patients, and to read the room for emotional and psychodynamic cues that may be affecting our ability to communicate effectively. All clinicians can take steps to enhance these capacities and thus show a fuller range of empathy for the patient. Curiosity and emotional intelligence are a good place to start.

Curiosity

Communication takes on real depth when it comes from a place of deep intention. If we are truly curious about patients' stories, that will come through in how we explore their experiences. Rather than hearing a clinician's prompts as, for example, a series of rapid-fire penetrating questions, the patient will see a caregiver across from them who is seeking connection and understanding. Ask yourself, "What might be motivating this patient's behavior?" or "What about this person's life do I not know, and how might that help me care for them better?" If you come from this place, you open up the possibility of learning extraordinary things. And, more importantly, you will always be authentic in your history taking.

In a similar way, we've also found that how we bring our personal stories into the room can powerfully affect our abilities as clinicians. Rachel Remen observed that clinicians who are attuned to their own stories can be surprised and moved. This possibility is one of the things that keep our curiosity alive. Many clinicians who deal with serious illness on a regular basis stay in this work for very personal reasons. These reasons, we find, usually take the form of stories – a story about how you made a difference, about what you found rewarding, about the change you wanted to make in the world. Every day, you are writing these stories, and within them, you can find a way to remind yourself about what part of yourself you want to bring forward.

As an example of this, palliative care consultants frequently care for patients with devastating neurological injuries whose families are trying to decide the best course forward, including whether to withhold hydration and nutrition. As it turns out, this was exactly the position that James and his family were in after his mother suffered a massive stroke. He knows what it's like to get consensus among a group of siblings, make a decision, and then have to fend off aggressive requests from relatives that don't have the full picture. That experience enters the room with him every time he sees such a patient and generates the deep empathy he feels for families facing this dilemma. He's never shared this story with a single family – there is no need to insert one's life so directly into a clinical encounter. However, his experience and feelings augment his curiosity and enable connection.

Emotional Intelligence

Our emotions tend to leak into our speech and, even more perniciously, our nonverbal behaviors. Notice, for example, the frustration (or even anger) you glimpse when a clinician says "As I've told you before." Emotional intelligence is the ability to understand and manage your own emotions, as well as to recognize and respond appropriately to the emotions of those around you. It's been described as consisting of five components: self-awareness, self-regulation, internal motivation, empathy, and social skills.

Emotional intelligence enables us to detect our emotions in real time and to manage them. This isn't just about self-control or feeling better. Being in touch with our own emotions can provide data that makes us better clinicians and builds more therapeutic relationships. For example, you may sense a patient's hopelessness because you are feeling hopeless yourself. This moment of shared futility can be turned into a moment of companionship and deep understanding. Although many of us learned in training that emotions are messy liabilities, we've come to appreciate that emotional intelligence, once acquired, gives us a whole additional realm of data that we use to understand other people. Not paying attention to our own internal emotional cues only makes communication with patients that much more difficult.

The better you get at communication skills, the more you need your emotional intelligence. For example, when you do a better job demonstrating empathy with your words, your patients will respond by disclosing more suffering, which in turn may trigger a reaction from you. So, as you improve in how you to talk to patients, expect to be challenged in this domain.

Developing the capacity to read your own emotions and then deal with them is beyond the scope of this book. But we can say this: it's worth every minute of time you invest. We've spent a lot of time figuring out how we're feeling after a tough conversation, how our own emotions influence what we say (and don't say), and how we can use our own emotions in a positive, healing way. We've sought out colleagues we trust, we've found good therapists, and we've gotten lots of feedback from people (clinicians, patients, and our families) whose judgment we trust. What we realize now is that the clinicians we really admire, who are extraordinary communicators and healers, have all done this kind of work – without exception.

FEEDBACK THAT CHANGED ME

I had been noticing that I had trouble with patients who frustrate me, but I was not sure why. One day I was rounding with our psychologist when it happened again: the patient started to frustrate me; I tried to be very polite, but she just got angrier. After the encounter, I asked the psychologist what she noticed. She observed that when frustrated, I talked slower – in an attempt to be hyper-polite. She hypothesized that the patient felt this was condescending. Now, when I am feeling angry and frustrated, I intentionally pay particular attention to how fast I am speaking and try to maintain a normal conversational rhythm. Patients no longer get angrier!

Expect Plateaus and Bad Days

What we haven't said yet is that improvement does not feel continuous. Many of us were raised with the assumption that learning is a continuous upward spiral of knowledge and glory. But, we've suggested that learning communication is akin to working on a sport skill. Anyone who has ever been coached on their tennis swing or golf stroke knows that undoing a habit, however unproductive, may make your overall game worse for a while. As you try to use your new communication skills, you may find that talking to patients suddenly becomes a bit more awkward. Unlearning old habits takes some attention, and energy. Progress in communication skills feels nonlinear, with some backsteps, sidesteps, and rough patches – but your patients will tell you as you're improving.

Be kind to yourself when you're having a bad day. When you are stressed or tired, you may revert to your old habits. Not a problem: this is normal. Leave behind the self-recrimination, the catastrophizing thoughts ("I'll never get this!"), and the self-pity. Just get back to your practice. If you are motivated, you can improve – and you'll get to where you use your skills instinctively. You'll gain more confidence, you'll improvise and riff, and you'll own it. Other people will think you were born this way.

Despite your skills, you may still occasionally run into the "patient from hell." We've all met someone who made us a little crazy. For example, one of us was once asked what to say to a patient who insisted on having his body sent into outer space as a kind of treatment. We did not have a good answer for this problem. Take a deep breath and remember that no one is perfect.

Taking Care of Yourself

We are living in an epidemic of clinician burnout. And for those of us who focus on the care of the seriously ill, the numbers may even be worse. Clinicians feel less in control, and stresses from the rest of the world, like racism and societal polarization, bleed into our practice. The COVID-19 pandemic raised the heat on a kettle that was already just below the boiling point. And, on top of all that, changes in practice, such as telehealth, risk reducing the joy many of us experience in our work through in-person, human connection. The risk is great. Burned-out clinicians don't communicate well, and poor communication leads to dissatisfied patients, which only compounds the problem. In the face of so many challenges, we cannot be passive. Clinicians need to actively seek meaning in their work and identify the resources that help to develop resiliency.

We hope that improving your communication skills is part of the solution. Better communication leads to more engaged clinical encounters, which help us remember why we went into this profession in the first place. Also, tasks such as delivering serious news and discussing goals of care can generate considerable anxiety for many clinicians. One tough conversation, particularly if it doesn't go well, can affect the whole rest of your day. If you have developed high-level skills that help you navigate these difficult conversations smoothly, you'll stop dreading them and feel more relaxed.

We also encourage you to develop other practices that build resilience. Placing boundaries around work and investing in the people you love is essential. Find passions outside of medicine and explore your spiritual life. Many clinicians find that maintaining a consistent meditation practice for as little as 20 minutes a day can be enormously grounding. Do whatever works for you, but make sure you do it.

What Does Mastery Look Like: What Are You Aiming For?

Once you develop a critical mass of skills, your conversations change in ways that are immediately noticeable to patients – and your colleagues. One course attendee emailed us days after returning home and practicing her new skills in clinic. She told us that her first patient of the day looked up at her and said, gratefully, "No one has ever talked to me like this." It was a deeply rewarding moment for that physician, and we know from experience that this can happen to you. These skills stick over the long run because you will get a lot of positive feedback from using them.

The Olympic-level communicators we know have lots of different communication tools, and they know how to use them. At the same time, they also have distinctively different styles, reflecting their personalities. Some are funny, others more serious, but like elite pole vaulters using different vaulting styles, they all clear the bar successfully. They are prepared for many different situations and are astute observers of what happens in a clinical encounter. Research on learning shows that experts see situations quite differently from novices. The experts notice different details, have larger and more extensive networks of knowledge, and can use their knowledge and observational power in a specific context. All this rings true for communication.

Furthermore, the most accomplished communicators can make it seem like there are no roadmaps at all. Having read this book, you will be able to identify much of what they do. But these elite communicators go beyond the roadmaps, and this leads us to an important caveat about this book. The roadmaps in this book are a scaffold for learning: they are intended to prop you up until you get your own foundation settled. After a while, you may no longer need them, just as scaffolding is taken down when the building is finished. Jerome Groopman wrote about finding individual metaphors to use with patients – a beautiful example of how communication can go beyond the roadmaps.

Finally, expert communicators bring something else into their clinical encounters. They have a way of putting every patient at the center of their attention, and a kind of ease with themselves. Whatever you call this quality – Rachel Remen talks about "presence," Carl Rogers labeled it "congruence," Howard Brody calls it a "healer's power" – it is immediately obvious, and probably not something you can learn from reading a book. But we point it out because it remains the hallmark of a clinical encounter in which a clinician can bring together biomedical expertise and a refined attentiveness to the whole person.

The Bottom Line

Mastery requires building both skills and capacities, practicing regularly, and caring for oneself in the process. And getting there will feel nonlinear, more like a series of small breakthroughs than a smooth continuous process. We hope (and believe) that when you arrive at that point, your patients will benefit from experiencing a clinician who truly heals, and you will derive deeper meaning and satisfaction from your professional practice.

Further Reading

Balint, M., *The Doctor, His Patient, and the Illness*. Churchill Livingstone, New York, 2000.

Bransford, J., A. L. Brown, and R. R. Cocking, eds., *How People Learn: Brain, Mind, Experience, and School*. National Academy Press, Washington, DC, 2000.

Childers, J. W., R. M. Arnold, and E. C. Carey, Striving and thriving: Challenges and opportunities for clinician emotional well-being. In Schwartz, R., J. A. Hall, and L.G. Osterberg, eds., *Emotion in the Clinical Encounter*. McGraw Hill, New York City, 2021.

Goleman, D., *Social Intelligence: The New Science of Human Relationships*. Bantam Books, New York, 2007.

Groopman, J., *The Measure of Our Days: A Spiritual Exploration of Illness*. London, Penguin, 1998.

Hunter, K., *Doctors' Stories: The Narrative Structure of Medical Knowledge*. Princeton University Press, Princeton, 1993.

Leiter, M. P. and C. Maslach, *Banishing Burnout: Six Strategies for Improving Your Relationship with Work*. Jossey-Bass, San Francisco, 2005.

Platt, F. W. and G. H. Gordon, *Field Guide to the Difficult Patient Interview. Field Guide Series*. Lippincott Williams & Wilkins, Philadelphia, 2004.

Silverman, J., S. M. Kurtz, and J. Draper, *Skills for Communicating with Patients*. Abingdon, Radcliffe Publishing, 2004.

Index